SECRETS

—— OF THE ——

17TH CENTURY
MEDICINE
CABINET

Katherine Knight trained as a teacher of home economics before getting married and bringing up her four children. She ran a poetry writing club at the City Lit, Holborn, for many years and has now expanded an interest in the history of cookery with the history of domestic medicine. She is the author of *The Mother and Daughter Cookbook* and *The Poet's Kit*. She lives in Strawberry Hill.

SECRETS

OF THE

17TH CENTURY

MEDICINE

CABINET

KATHERINE KNIGHT

The History Press

For Daniel, Amy and Helen

Cover illustrations from the Wellcome Collection.

First published 2006 as *How Shakespeare Cleaned His Teeth and Cromwell Treated His Warts*
This paperback edition first published 2024

The History Press
97 St George's Place, Cheltenham,
Gloucestershire, GL50 3QB
www.thehistorypress.co.uk

British Library Cataloguing in Publication Data.
A catalogue record for this book is available from the British Library.

ISBN 978 1 80399 701 8

Typesetting and origination by The History Press
Printed and bound in Great Britain by TJ Books Limited, Padstow, Cornwall.

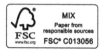

Trees for LYfe

Contents

Acknowledgements

This book is based on an article which won the Folklore Society's McDowall Prize, 2001, for an essay on a folklore topic written by an author unconnected with an academic institution. An extract from this was published in *Folklore*, Vol. 113, No. 2, 2002, to which grateful acknowledgement is made.

Thanks also for generous help given by the following people:

Dr Richard Aspin, Curator of Western Manuscripts, The Wellcome Institute, and his staff, who made suggestions for further reading and provided background information on the domestic manuscripts I used.

Anne Stobart, Nicky Wesson and other members of the Medical Receipts Research Group for stimulating discussions, and Susan Drury for allowing me access to her unpublished M. Phil. thesis.

Karen Howell, Curator, The Old Operating Theatre Museum and Herb Garret, Southwark, for answering several herbal and historical questions.

James Robinson, Curator of Medieval Collections, Department of Prehistory and Europe, The British Museum, and Dr Silke Ackermann, for showing me their collection of magical amulets and rings, and making suggestions for more research.

But, notwithstanding all this, any mistakes that remain are my very own.

A Note on Weights
and Measures

The weights and measures of the seventeenth century bore a
family resemblance to our own pre-metric ones, but two sys-
tems were in use.

The older standard of Troy weight still applied to precious
metals, gemstones and apothecaries' drugs; the avoirdupois system
to many other things.

Gideon Harvey, in his book *The Family Physician and the House
Apothecary*, has a helpful table to tell his readers what was what, at
least in 1676. The basic unit was the grain, that is a grain of corn,
which goes back to Roman times as the smallest unit of weight.

WEIGHTS

A Physical [medical] Pound (which is Troy *weight) contains only twelve
ounces.*

The Druggists and Grocers Pound (being Aver de poiz *weight) contains
sixteen ounces.*

*An Ounce contains eight Drams. A Dram contains three Scruples. A
Scruple contains twenty Grains.*

MEASURES

A Pint measure in most watery Liquors, weighs twelve ounces. Two Quarts make a Pottle, two Pottles make a Gallon.

A Fascicle signifies an Armful. One Handful is as much as a moderate hand can take up. A Pugil is as much as you can take up with your Thumb and two next Fingers.

It may be noted that the Pint in this table is much less than the Imperial standard pint, 20 fluid oz, of recent memory. There may be less liquid therefore in the receipts than might be thought at first reading, provided the writers were using Gideon Harvey's pint.

Mrs Miller, in Wellcome MS 3547 (1660), gave the same number of grains, scruples and drams to the ounce at the start of her book.

Foreword

Anyone caught up in the recent Covid pandemic ought to sympathise with victims of historical plagues. For instance, in 1665 entire families could be quarantined for forty days, locked down in their homes. Many died.

Even in more normal times access to seventeenth-century health care was patchy. When the Tudor monasteries were closed, most of their attached hospitals had been shut down with them. Academic physicians were scarce and expensive. Apothecaries, who sold medicines, were frequently their antagonistic rivals. Ideas about sickness were still based on classical writers such as Galen.

Herbs were the main sources of effective drugs. Traditional country lore was often helpful, though mixed with magic and superstition. Nursing the sick and supplying cures depended mostly on the family, local priest or village midwife. Notebooks kept by housewives show a very interesting mixture of remedies, rather like our internet, some useful, some problematic. These notebooks are the basis of this book.

Things were changing, though, especially in the later part of the century. The Royal Society, under the patronage of Charles II, included members starting to apply scientific method to the investigation of disease. The development of the microscope revealed a whole new world, hitherto invisible.

Most of the contents of the seventeenth-century medicine cabinet are now long past their use-by date. But we can understand why

they were there. They were part of the continuing human search
for longer, healthier lives.

Katherine Knight,
February 2024

Introduction

I came across seventeenth-century household medicine by lucky chance. I had been interested in cookery history for many years, and when I discovered that the Wellcome Library had a number of unpublished household manuscripts dating from early modern times I went to look at them.

What I found was fascinating. It is easy to sympathise with people noting down recipes for such things as pies, stews and preserves. Making allowance for differences in kitchen equipment, these cooks seem very much like ourselves in period dress. But mixed with the food, there were many recipes – or 'receipts' as they were then known – for a multitude of remedies which could be made at home. The diseases treated would nowadays send us rushing off to the nearest hospital: consumption, bladder stone, plague and frenzy, for instance. While the cookery in these manuscripts reveals a reasonably familiar kitchen, the medicine shows a far stranger place, where plants understandably provide most of the drugs available, but where magic can easily bubble up out of ancient traditions.

I wondered how representative these examples were, and went on to compare them with printed sources. The printed books were a little more literate, as might be expected. But there wasn't much to choose between the presumably more 'official' printed books and the manuscripts. Indeed, there was evidence of borrowing between them in both directions, and the printed books had their full share of extraordinary and magical ingredients. If some of the medicines were by our standards barbaric, it was not a simple case of primitive survivals in manuscripts alone.

The compilers of the manuscript collections obviously invested a lot of effort in producing them. They give a general impression of being meant for use, not made for fun. Some were written by several people, occasionally by succeeding generations. But the writers were not critical of what they wrote. Cures which must have been old-fashioned or superstitious even in the seventeenth century were put down pell-mell with sensible herbal medicines, cookery recipes, the family doctor's recommendations, and items from books and friends. There is little to show whether the remedies were really effective or not, apart from the *probatum est*, or 'approved', sometimes added even to far-fetched items.

There may well be valuable medicine to be rediscovered from old receipts such as these, and especially from oral traditions of country cures. Some plant-drugs have indeed entered the modern pharmacopoeia, such as senna, aspirin from willow bark, and an extract of yew to help cancer.

Caution

These receipts are offered for their historical interest, and certainly not for modern use. While some herbal remedies are highly effective they can also be highly poisonous. If they are used at all the dosage must be carefully monitored by an expert. Besides, the herbal plants mentioned may not be the same as the ones in use today. There may be a confusion of names, particularly common names found in different parts of the country.

Some receipts are disgusting, and some involve cruelty to animals. Home distillation of alcohol is illegal and dangerous. Although the good housewife and seventeenth-century physicians were doing their best, there are several reasons why expectation of life is generally longer today!

But the receipts offer a moving glimpse of family life in the seventeenth century, the worries of parents about their children, the suffering that could occur at any moment, and optimism, too. Theories of disease seem to have been left mostly to the academic physicians. The housewife was concerned with practical matters.

This book then is partly about the skills of the home practitioner, and so belongs to domestic social history. It is also a representative collection of seventeenth-century receipts, part of the story of English medicine. But I have also tried to account for some of the more extraordinary ingredients that were used, so it is a book of folklore, too. It shows people like ourselves struggling with health problems, doing their best to cure themselves. If their methods and assumptions often seem strange, they came just before the starting-point for modern discoveries. To look at them is like looking at a family album of faded sepia photographs, where great-great-grandma sits on an uncomfortable chair, with great-great-grandpa unsmiling behind her. They are alien, and yet our kin.

I

The Stuart Housewife
and Household Books

The Good Wife

Superwoman is timeless. She was illuminated in medieval manuscripts, harvesting in fields, milking cows, working in kitchens, busy in child-bed and sick-bed scenes. By the seventeenth century she was even more documented, caring for family and home, standing-in for a husband away at war, helping him in business as an extension of her home duties, or continuing as a widow. It was expected that most girls would become wives and mothers (or servants), with unremitting physical labour. A very few aristocratic ladies had independent interests, in neighbourhood medicine or writing for example, and others became courtesans. But for most, the honourable work of the housewife was normal. Without her, there was no comfort for anyone.

Gervase Markham, whose book *The English Hous-wife*, intended for 'anie compleat Hous-wife of what degree or calling soever', was first published in 1615 and went into several expanded editions after that. The woman's skills included physic, i.e. medicine, cookery, organising banquets, distillation, treatment of wool, hemp, and flax, dairy work, brewing, baking, and everything else expected in a household. She was meant to be religious, temperate, dressed decently in clean garments, moderate in diet and full of general virtues such as courage, patience and discretion. She was expected to have a pleasant manner, so the household would run harmoniously.[1]

Home-doctoring had to be fitted in with many other things, but depending on her social position, she would have some help. A woman who was truly proficient in all the skills recommended by Markham was not only a considerable craftswoman, but needed managerial and teaching ability to get the best out of her servants. These servants were comparatively plentiful, but needed supervision, as they were often very young.

To start with, the task of clothing a family in the country meant a choice of wool or linen fabric. Imported silk and Indian cotton could be bought in the towns, but cotton did not supersede traditional fabrics for some time. To get good, hard-wearing woollen cloth the fleeces had to be cleaned, dyed, oiled, carded and spun. The spinning wheel had been introduced to Europe in the Middle Ages, a labour-saving mechanism better than the old distaff and spindle, but even so spinning was an occupation taken up whenever nothing more urgent had to be done. Weaving was a specialist craft, but the sewing of everyday clothes was part of most women's life. Turning flax into linen, and linen into shirts, sheets, table-cloths and napkins was a similar process. Embroidered fabrics were luxuries. Once made, clothes were valued, and looked after as carefully as possible.

Most food was produced locally, because transportation was expensive and slow, and perishable foodstuffs would go bad on long journeys. Butter and cheese were made from raw milk for consumption in the household, or sent to a nearby market. Milk had to be processed quickly, especially in hot weather. Brewing was a business open to women, though many households made their own beer and ale rather than buying it in. It was an important task. Water might be contaminated, and it was preferable, even for children, to drink ale or beer. Wine was imported in large quantities for the rich, and was used medicinally, as well.

Cookery was obviously of great value, and to feed the family properly every dish had to be prepared from basic ingredients, which came mostly from the farm, garden, or neighbourhood market. Some commodities, such as sugar, spices, almonds and olive oil, were imported, as they had been through the Middle Ages, but compared to local produce they were expensive luxuries. Luxurious, too, was the 'banquetting stuff'. The banquet was a separate course, or perhaps an after-dinner party might be a better description. Upper-class families even had separate buildings for the banquet. Elaborate sweets were made from marchpane (marzipan), fruit pastes and sugar-plate. The production of these things was somewhere between art and cookery. You could for instance make sugar-plate coloured and flavoured with flowers.[2] Bread might be made by the village baker, but here again a large household might produce its own.

Distillation covered both the making of medicines and cordials from such things as fruit and flowers, and the perfumes that must have added much to the pleasure of home. In the absence of piped water, washing was far more difficult and less frequent, though people still liked to be clean according to the standards of the time. Sanitation was similarly rudimentary.

All this meant that the housewife needed a great deal of stoicism as well as stamina. There were the usual natural disasters to cope with – sickness of all kinds including plague, and irregularities in food supply due to bad harvests. It was normal to have many pregnancies, and common to lose infants. It has been estimated that an average of 160 babies out of every 1,000 born alive did not reach their first birthday.[3] This proportion was higher in the unhealthy towns. In the middle of the century, the Civil War added its horrors and losses. Many men died of battle wounds or disease, leaving widows and orphans. Food was often commandeered by soldiers, and destruction of property added to hardship. Even modest houses could be ruined, as well as grander aristocratic establishments.

It is difficult to generalise about the literacy of women. Some girls were taught to read, and privileged ones were educated alongside their brothers at home, but women were not admitted to universities. There were a few schools for ordinary people, but in general girls were taught domestic skills rather than intellectual ones, though running a large household demanded high intelligence. It was of course only comparatively well-educated women who were able to keep household books of recipes and medicines. As so many survive, it may indicate that more women were being better taught as the century progressed, but men too were involved in writing some of the receipts.

HOUSEHOLD BOOKS

These manuscripts give a real sense of different personalities. They are varied in style, some written by several people, some in a single hand. They may be neat, perhaps prepared by young girls to take with them into marriage, while others are more slapdash with blots and cancellations. Over time, a number of people might contribute: perhaps a daughter and granddaughter continuing a notebook which they had inherited. Several have cookery and medical receipts set down without organisation. For instance, in 1699 a cure for urinary gravel appears between recipes for potted tongue and potted herrings. Plum porridge, surfeit water and 'a Good Baked puding' are close neighbours.[4] Generally the printed books, like Gervase Markham's, are easier to consult, being divided into sections. A few manuscripts notebooks have cookery recipes at one end, medical ones at the other. Others are devoted entirely to medicines, or as we would say now, treatments. They include such things as poultices and glisters (enemas), not just preparations to be swallowed. Though some appear to be written by comparatively humble people, even the humblest had to be more or less literate. The social range is from roughly middle class to the élite. A few simple country remedies are recorded here and there.

At the top of the range, one beautifully written medical book was owned and used by the Countess of Arundel in her charitable work. A substantial book, about 22 cm by 16 cm, now bound in brown leather, it has written on the flyleaf '*Liber Comitissae Arundeliae* A Booke of divers Medicines Broothes, salves Waters, Syropps and Oyntementes of w[hi]ch many or the most part have been experienced and tryed by the special practize of Mrs Corlyon. Anno D'ni 1606.' It has been suggested that it was a presentation copy to be given as a wedding present.[5] Three copies are known, the one at the Wellcome Library, MS 213, one in the Folger Library, New York, and one at Arundel Castle. It is written in a very clear hand. Red ink was used for the headings, or to mark an important new step in directions. There are very few mistakes. It is divided into logical chapters and has a table of contents. The Wellcome copy has a few additions in a different hand. It was still being used at the end of the seventeenth century, described as 'a great treasure', and formed part of the recent exhibition of Henry Wellcome's collection, *Medicine Man*, in the British Museum (2003). I must admit that handling this bound manuscript, produced when Shakespeare was still alive, made me feel very close to the person writing it. There was obvious pride in the craftsmanship.

In less formal collections, even in a few printed examples, cookery and medical receipts seem to be noted as they cropped up, with a sprinkling of household hints such as how to make sealing wax and keep your poultry safe from weasels, by rubbing them over with rue. The pocket-book 'written partly by Edw[ar]d Kidder & par[t]ly by Kath[e]r[in]e Kidder' already mentioned and dated 1699, was of this kind. There are, for instance, directions to make 'Little Courons Cake', followed by 'A Most excelent Bath for the Goute or lameness by salte humers',[6] which was made from boiled herbs, 'a large quantity of urin and a good large quantity of ston hors Dung, boiled together'. You put this in a wooden tub and sat with your legs in it up to the knees for an hour a day, for 10 days. 'It will sartainly Qure the goute though in the hands or arms as well as leggs onely by sitting in it.' (Horse dung was used as a gentle source of heat for many purposes.) Then, having climbed out of the tub, you got on with the next receipts, 'To preserve Cheryes in Jelly', 'The Green Oyntment', a magic spell to cure ague, and 'To make surrop of vilotts'. This is Wellcome MS 3107, Kidder.

Even more interesting perhaps is the book of *Select Receipts, 'taken out of Lady Barretts Bookcase ... 1711'* with the name 'Ann Egerton' above a book plate. Internal evidence suggests it was started some time after 1648 (Wellcome MS 1071, Barrett). It is about the same size as a chunky Filofax. It consists of medical receipts only, in several hands. The first of these is small, neat and literate, written by F. Head – many of the receipts are initialled 'F. H.' and he refers to 'Grandmother Head' at one point. This is certainly a man, as he refers to his wife. The second important contributor, probably a woman, initialled her work 'H. S.' Both these people utilise archaic material, so one can't draw conclusions about a more enlightened male or female compiler.

There are many other collections in the Wellcome Library, among which are a small book, written on vellum now dark with age, signed inside the front cover *Grace Acton, May 1621* (Wellcome MS 1); and *A Book of Receipts* by Mrs Jane Baber, 1625 (MS 108), a frail unbound one. Many people had an input into *Cookery and medical receipts 1636–47, Townsend Family Papers* (MS 774); the size of a school exercise book. *Mrs Jane Parker her Booke Anno 1651* (MS 3769) is an example of a notebook started from both ends, with cookery and medical receipts reversed. A rather later household book is *Mrs Mary Miller her Booke of Receipts 1660* (MS 3547), a fairly scruffy manuscript 20 cm x 15 cm, written in many hands, with cookery recipes first, medical ones later. Many pages have been left blank, to leave space for additions. The content is similar to those written earlier in the period.

Published works, many written by men for the use of women, were useful to supplement and compare with my research, particularly Gervase Markham's book. Mrs Corlyon's manuscript book can be studied alongside *With Faith and Physic, The Life of a Tudor Gentlewoman: Lady Grace Mildmay 1552–1620* (published 1993). The pious Lady Mildmay was an unofficial medical practitioner, and this book gives many of her receipts as well as devotions. Robert Burton's *Anatomy of Melancholy*, of 1621, has much to say about medicine in general and emotional problems in particular.

Another useful one is *The Good Housewife's Jewel* by Thomas Dawson, 1596. Mostly cookery, it also contains a short chapter on husbandry, including a humoral treatment for apple trees. The medical section has forty receipts. A small book in black-letter type, *The Treasvrie of Hidden Secrets*, 1637, was clearly written for women, as it contains a lot of obstetric lore – though of an old-fashioned kind. It also has practical housekeeping tips, cookery and general medical receipts. Later a handbook written by Jane Sharp, a practising midwife, describes her craft and its lore in 1671.

A Mr W. M. who claimed he had been a servant of Queen Henrietta Maria, published a work in three sections under the blanket title of *The Queen's Closet Opened*. The first part is medical, *The Pearl of Practice*. The second, *The Compleat Cook*, is concerned with cookery, and the third, *A Queens Delight*, has to do with conserving, distilling and so on, and covers both preserves and medicinal waters. It was first published in 1655 and went through many editions, remaining popular until 1713. He said he had decided to publish the authentic work only because someone else had started to bring it out without authority. Echoing this title is *The Closet of the Eminently Learned Sir Kenelme Digbie Kt. Opened*. A closet was a small private room, which often contained curios. It hints at secrets being revealed. Sir Kenelm was a Royalist courtier, traveller, linguist and one of the founder-members of The Royal Society. His book, published posthumously in 1669, was put together by an assistant, George Hartman. It is a compendium of receipts for mead, metheglin, cider and fruit wines, plus potages, savoury and sweet dishes, with only an occasional nod in the direction of physic. It gives a good idea of the attitudes to meat and drink of an aristocrat of the time, a kind of early foodie.

A later book, *The Gentlewoman's Companion, Or, A Guide to the Female Sex*, 1675, is attributed to Hannah Woolley, an experienced writer of cookery books. This one is primarily concerned with social duties and etiquette, including letter-writing, perhaps for the upwardly mobile. It contains guides for servants – cooks, dairymaids, chamber-maids and others, and a small section of about three dozen medical receipts. It demonstrates how generally static household remedies remained through the period.

Herbals were available too, not only describing plants but giving medical directions for their use. The most famous of these is John Gerarde's *Herball, or Generall Historie of Plantes*, 1597. Gerarde was in charge of a physic garden belonging to the College of Physicians. Possibly even more influential for poorer people after the Civil War was Nicholas Culpeper's *The English Physitian* which first appeared in 1652. Many editions followed, and it is still in print. Culpeper had previously been responsible for translating the official pharmacopoeia, the 1618 *Pharmacopoeia Londinensis* of the College of Physicians, from Latin into English, so that ordinary people could treat themselves. The translation, with the title *A Physical Directory*, was published for the first time in 1649, and because it attempted to break the monopoly of the physicians, they did not like it at all. Culpeper, who had trained as an apothecary, did not like the physicians much either, and added acerbic comments of his own.

For those traditionalists who harked back to classical learning, but could not study the original in Latin, there was a translation of Pliny's *Natural History* made by Philemon Holland and published in 1601. Those who could read Latin could go back to versions of the classics, of course, and so perpetuate venerable ideas.

MEDICINE IN THE HOME

Those who could not afford the high fees of a licensed physician had to rely on home care, and that usually meant women's work. Markham acknowledged that looking after the family's health was a very important part of the housewife's duty:

> To beginne then with one of the most principall vertues which doth belong to our English hous-wife; you shall understand that sith the preseruation and care of the familie touching their health and sound-nesse of bodie consisteth most in her diligence: it is meet that shee haue a phisicall [medical] kinde of knowledge; how to administer many wholsome receits or medicines for the good of their healthes, as well to preuent the first occasion of sicknesse, as to take away the effects and euill of the same when it hath made seazure on the body.

However, she had to be careful not to usurp the place of a proper, learned physician, who had spent much time at University, and was thoroughly educated in classical theories of disease. As in religion, she should defer to established authority. Her intellect was inferior. 'Indeed we must confesse that the depth and secrets of this most excellent art of phisicke, is farre beyond the capacitie of the most skilful weoman, as lodging only in the brest of the learned Professors; yet ... our hous-wife may from them receiue some ordinary rules, and medicines ...'[7]

Cookery and kitchen physic were still closely allied. Good food, fresh and naturally produced, was then, as now, accepted as necessary for good health, though dietetics followed the theories of Galen, which in turn depended on the theory of humours (see p. 27). The

Middle Ages had added some prejudices of its own, such as the idea that fresh fruit could cause 'flux'. To be fair, though, this was very possibly true if the water used for irrigation was polluted. The first cookery treatise in English, *The Forme of Cury*, which dates from 1399, claimed to be written with the help of 'masters of physic and of philosophy'. 'A good coke is halfe a physycyon,' said Dr Andrew Boorde famously, during the reign of Henry VIII.

From Elizabethan times, middle-class and noble households possessed a lot of kitchen equipment, and there were separate still-rooms for making luxuries such as conserves, candies, perfumes, cosmetics and cordials. Sir Hugh Plat's *Delightes for Ladies, to adorne their Persons, Tables, Closets and Distillatories with Beauties, Banquets, Perfumes & Waters* was published in 1609, though it contains only a few medical recipes. But the equipment could well be used to produce hundreds of 'waters', mostly based on herbs, spices and wine.

PROVENANCE OF RECEIPTS

Although the Galenic system was reformed in the later seventeenth century, traditional treatments lingered on alongside pragmatic remedies. Some items appear to come directly from practical experience – using mashed onion to dress a burn for instance, credited to 'Mrs Gregorie.' in the Barrett manuscript.[8] Even so it may have originated from a printed herbal.

Many go back a very long way. Pliny, Dioscorides and Galen might describe a remedy using a certain herb or animal part, and it would then persist by copying and translation through the ages, with change of language and some modification, but basically the same identity. Receipts once given shape in writing were difficult to dislodge. For instance, the little Acton manuscript (itself dated 1621), contains both cookery and medical recipes, and the cookery ones are certainly medieval. 'Browet of Almayne', 'viande royal', 'Boar in egreduce' are the same recipes that appear in *The Forme of Cury*, mentioned above. It isn't unreasonable to suppose, then, that the medical entries are also of great age, circumstantial evidence for thinking that medical receipts might be handed down through household books for hundreds of years. On the other hand, mention of gunpowder or tobacco proves a more or less contemporary source for some of the cures elsewhere.

There was also an exchange of receipts and ideas between friends. Just as today people collect recipes – 'Do tell me how you made this delicious mango sorbet!' – so medical receipts were part of the same social exchange, then copied and perhaps passed on again. The originator was often acknowledged, especially if an aristocrat or doctor. Mrs Corlyon has many such: 'A Medecine for the Rhewme in the teethe or Gummes taughte by Mrs Maynarde', 'A Medecine for the Coughe ... La: Russell,' and 'A Plaister prescribed by Dr Foster' are just three examples.[9]

Some items were undoubtedly taken from published sources. Thus 'Dr Stevens' water' is given by Markham.[10] An almost identical recipe, using many of the same phrases, is included in Barrett,[11] plus a shortened version. Parker has a celebrated cure for the plague which the Lord Mayor (presumably of London), was said to have received from the Queen herself.[12] A similar cure appears in *The Queen's Closet Opened*, of 1655, though perhaps from a source common to both. Mrs Corlyon has a much praised plaster, 'Paracelsus his plaister called Implastrum Fodicationum Paracelsi, good for many diseases mentioned vndernethe'[13] which turns up, almost word for word, in *The Queen's Closet* again[14] though ounces have been changed to drams.

It is easy to imagine Markham's ideal housewife having just finished some entries in her book after a hard day's work in nursery, kitchen, dairy, still-room and garden.

She wiped her inky quill on a rag, and sat still for a rare moment's rest. Her sister had just written to her from London with a wonderful new receipt for an ointment using tobacco, and the latest way to preserve pippins. She had added this information to her notebook, together with directions for making invisible ink and a cordial water which would use up the glut of strawberries in the garden.

She was thinking not only about her immediate family but of her servants, neighbours and friends, as well. Little Betty had a worrying cough. The old carpenter in the village had shrunken sinews, and one of the maids had burnt her hand with hot grease in the kitchen yesterday. But her garden was full of delightful and useful herbs. She was lucky her mother had left her so many good recipes, and had taught her to read and write. Her book was a treasure to her. Some diseases were difficult to manage, but at least she could fill her cupboards with rare waters and soothing ointments. With God's help the patients might recover.

She sighed. It was getting dark and she didn't want to waste candles. She closed the book, but she would certainly open it again tomorrow.

2

Background to
17th-Century Medicine

The seventeenth century was an exciting time for well-educated and enquiring men, provided they could negotiate religious fanaticism, political power struggles and the Civil War, and survive the various plagues and fevers which surrounded them. By the end of the century, Natural Philosophy covered wide fields of enquiry, from astronomy, on a large scale, to microscopy, on a very small one. Alchemy flowed from a distant past to a golden future after it was transmuted into chemistry. With hindsight, we can see that 'science' was not a new concept. For example, as far back as the thirteenth century Roger Bacon (*c*.1220–1292), had studied mathematics, optics and astronomy, as well as alchemy and languages. His work on the nature of light anticipated Newton. (The double-edged benefit of science was apparent even then: Bacon described both gunpowder and eyeglasses.) A later philosopher, coincidentally with the same name, proposed a method of inquiry depending on experiment and deductive reasoning. This was Francis Bacon (1561–1626). Many members of The Royal Society, founded after the Restoration of Charles II in 1660, picked up scientific method and ran with it into the modern world.

This was just at the top of the intellectual pyramid, however. Men of high social position were frequently sent off to University, either in Britain or abroad, but the rest of the population got by with far less learning. Adult male literacy was not universal. Women were even less likely to be educated. As far as medicine was concerned, physicians were still struggling to make it a profession of high status, like Law or the Church. As in those callings, medicine had to be based on authoritative texts to be academically acceptable. A physician's training since medieval times included liberal subjects such as rhetoric and mathematics besides classical theories of disease. Only the richest patients could consult these physicians, whose high standing was reflected in their fees. They were in competition with each other, and a person could go from one to another if he was dissatisfied with his cure.

For poorer people there were other ways of getting help without calling in an expensive doctor. You could ask for advice from your family, your neighbours or the parish priest. Some people went to the local wise woman with good results, though it was debatable if magical cures were legitimate. 'Sorcerers are too common; cunning men, wizards, and white witches, as they call them, in every village, which, if they be sought unto, will help almost all infirmities of body and mind,' said Robert Burton.[1] He concluded that it might be better to suffer than to be damned for meddling with the devil. Given this attitude, it is surprising that 'white witches' were kind enough to help anyone apart from their immediate and trusted family and neighbours. An accusation of witchcraft was serious and potentially fatal.

It was possible to find a quack with a miraculous panacea at the fair; or, in towns, to visit an apothecary or surgeon, who had received practical training. Surgery was generally regarded as an inferior craft, best left to artisans. Drugs such as opium, its derivative laudanum, mandrake and other narcotics were given as pain-killers, but they were themselves dangerous and surgery was limited in scope.

Most hospitals had been closed with the Dissolution of the Monasteries. Only a few, such as St. Bartholomew's, survived. Even serious diseases were treated at home, and recovery depended as much on careful nursing as anything else. A household book must have been a vital resource in trouble. Undoubtedly though, many of the receipts did come from physicians in the first place, though the compilers did not question the underlying ideas.

Nevertheless these ideas had had a long and interesting history.

HIPPOCRATES AND GALEN

Doctors' treatments, often claimed to be 'approved' or with the Latin equivalent *Probatum est* were used because they always had been. Right up to the seventeenth century, and even beyond, orthodox medicine lay on foundations of Hippocratic and Galenic theory.

Hippocrates of Cos was a legendary Greek doctor (*c.* 460–370 BC). In fact, about sixty different treatises make up the Hippocratic Corpus, gathered together in Alexandria in about 250 BC.[2] The normal state of a stable body was health. Disease resulted from a disruption of equilibrium. Various humours, or physical fluids, were constantly ebbing and flowing through the human system, and the aim of the doctor was to correct any imbalance. Galen later perfected and codified this theory.

Hippocratic medicine was holistic, full of common sense. It laid stress on leading a healthy life, rather than on battling against disease. Diet, exercise, sleep, bathing, and sex ought to be regulated according to one's temperament, stage of life, and the season. Geographical location was important – marshy areas were known to be unhealthy for example. Bad air was dangerous. Disease had natural causes, and was not inflicted by the gods. If changes in lifestyle didn't help, medicine might be given. Surgery was a last resort, and too dangerous for a physician to attempt. It was left to specialist craftsmen. Part of the Hippocratic Oath, which dates from somewhere between the fifth and third centuries BC,[3] says 'I will not cut, even for the stone, but I will leave such procedures to the practitioners of that craft.' The demarcation between physicians and surgeons was to persist up to modern times.

In contrast with the shadowy Hippocrates, Galen of Pergamon (129–216 AD), was a solid historical figure, though later regarded as almost superhuman. He was a well-educated and privileged Greek, the son of an architect. It was said that his father had a dream sent by the healing god Aesclepius, who gave instructions that the boy should become a doctor. Accordingly Galen studied at the best institutions of the time, and in 157 became a physician to gladiators in Pergamon. His experience of wounds, and hence physiology, was invaluable, and after a few years he went to Rome, to treat the wealthy there. He eventually became physician to several Roman Emperors. He was a philosopher as well as a doctor, carried out dissections on animals, and wrote extensively, with passion and logic. He promoted himself as perfecting the work started by Hippocrates. In fact his writings were so brilliant that they remained the best medical knowledge for more than a thousand years. He was so much respected that questioning his conclusions was a kind of heresy, and this held back progress as we define it. If a fact did not fit into Galen's system, it was assumed to be a false observation, or perhaps humanity had degenerated since his time. In Europe, bodies of executed criminals were used for rare dissections, so it was easy to suggest that they were abnormal anyway.

This was to change slowly during the Renaissance, but at first efforts to improve medicine aimed at correcting corrupt classical texts rather than testing theories in practice.

Anglo-Saxon Medicine

During the so-called Dark Ages, classical writings were saved and copied in centres of learning such as Bede's Northumbria. Medical texts came to be written in the Anglo-Saxon vernacular too, the *Lacnunga* manuscript and the *Leechbook of Bald* being the most famous.[4] ('*Laece*' was simply the Old English word for a healer.) These works represent a side step away from the classics to some extent. Although influenced by them, they contain some remedies based on what looks like practical knowledge recently discovered at that time.

The medicine is mostly herbal, but the remedies are much simpler than the later ones of the household books. There is much overt magic such as the use of charms and incantations. Nevertheless, there is a strong family resemblance to some of the receipts of the household manuscripts of the seventeenth century. Ingredients such as earthworms, several kinds of animal dung, foxes' grease and so on are common to both, and some in fact can be traced back to Pliny, Dioscorides and other classical authorities. It might be surmised that some of these old remedies persisted in folk culture through the Middle Ages, and fragments resurfaced into the manuscript household books.

Theories of disease differed from those of Galen. The body might be attacked from the outside by 'flying venom' for example, which caused epidemics, or by the magical elf-shot which brought sickness to animals, as well as complaints such as rheumatism to human beings. A worm might introduce poison and simultaneously remove vitality. 'Unhealth' was something which could be removed, perhaps by emetics. Ointments were applied to seal the body against external attacks and to preserve the positive health within it.[5]

MEDIEVAL (AND LATER) MEDICINE

During the early Middle Ages, medical care had largely been in the jurisdiction of the Church. Healing the sick was a part of its ministry. But there was an obligation on those in Holy Orders not to shed blood, so such men could not offer a complete medical package which included venesection. A lay technician was needed for routine bleeding. Surgery was not a high-status occupation. Increasingly there were lay physicians too, educated at the nascent faculties of medicine in Universities,such as Solerno. This one was particularly well-known to ordinary people because of its compilation of rules for health in the thirteenth century, *Regimen Sanitatis Salerni*. There were many translations, including one by the Elizabethan courtier, Sir John Harrington, who, incidentally, is supposed to have invented a flushing water-closet for the Queen.

The Crusades brought the existence of Arabic medicine to the attention of the West. This medicine was also based on classical texts of Hippocrates and Galen, but with the addition of advances made in Alexandria and later discoveries. Ibn Sina, known as Avicenna in the West (980–1037) is just one example of a celebrated physician. He produced a definitive *Canon* of medicine which became one of the set-books of the emerging Universities.

The persistent Galenic theory of humours taught that there were four main body fluids. It was a neat and satisfying system, connected to the four seasons, the four ages of human life – childhood, youth, maturity and old age – and above all the four Aristotelian elements of earth, air, fire and water. Thus black bile, or the melancholy humour, had an affinity with earth, blood with air, yellow bile or choler with fire , and phlegm with water. Elements and humours were assigned four qualities, hot, cold, moist and dry. Earth and black bile were dry and cold, air and blood were hot and moist. Fire and yellow bile were hot and dry, and finally water and phlegm were cold and moist. An excess of any humour resulted in a problem, but phlegm and black bile were especially troublesome. It was an elegant theory which seemed to give an explanation for many conditions.

All four humours were present in the body, but according to one's individual bias they gave rise to different 'complexions' or temperaments – melancholic, sanguine, choleric and phlegmatic. (We still use the same terms to describe different types of personality.) In the classical view, treatment had to be fitted to the patient's individual complexion, age, and so on. It was holistic medicine, treating the person, rather than seeing the disease as an invasive entity as we may do today. Even as late as 1676 a doctor could warn against unqualified mountebanks and their medicines, 'which being so indifferently and rashly used by many credulous persons, at all times and seasons, without that particular regard had to their Constitution, Age, Sex, Climate and Cause of Disease, must necessarily, if not kill, at least destroy the Temperament of their Bowels and noble parts.'[6] (This warning would have been more persuasive if physicians themselves had known more about the real Cause of Disease.)

It followed from this theory that an illness was cured by rebalancing the humours that were out of kilter with opposite qualities in food or medicine. If there was too much of one, it could be removed by various methods. Too much blood, a plethora, was corrected by the application of leeches which sucked blood, or by phlebotomy, where a vein was cut and allowed to flow before being bound up again.

There was a great emphasis on purging. Laxatives were given, and so were emetics to produce vomiting. The idea here was to remove excessive humours, venom or poison from the digestive system. Sweating would eliminate it through the skin.

A hot dry fever could be reduced by cold, moist medicine. Too much phlegm was controlled by hot and dry substances. Melancholy was rather more of a problem, as it frequently had what we would call a psychological component. It was often treated with purging. In practice the system was complex, as the age of the patient and the season had their effects as well. Even in the seventeenth century, some healers were still taking account of astrology too. Culpeper is an example.

Food, herbs and spices were assigned 'degrees' of heat, cold, dryness and moistness, which gave a reassuringly rational air to their medicinal use. The scale ran from the gentlest, 1, to 3, with 4 the impossibly pure and violent quality, usually unobtainable in practice. As an example, Culpeper's *Herbal* has this to say about cucumbers:

> ... they are so much cried out against for their coldness, and if they were but one degree colder they would be poison. The best of Galenists hold them to be cold and moist in the second degree ... they are excellent good for a hot stomach and hot liver; the unmeasurable use of them fills the body full of raw humours ...

Plants were the main source of medicines throughout antiquity, the Middle Ages and continued so to the eighteenth century, though other substances were used too, some in magical fashion. Even before Galen, herbalists listed the uses, or virtues, of common herbs and spices. One of the most influential was Dioscorides, a Greek surgeon in Nero's service in the first century AD. His book is generally called by its Latin title, *De materia medica*. It is an encyclopaedia of therapeutic substances, many of vegetable origin (herbs, roots, trees, seeds, wines ...) but including a number of animal parts and minerals. Their use in medicine was described, together with tips on gathering and storing. Such a useful book was copied and recopied right through the Middle Ages, often with illustrations added, though pictures became more symbolic than accurate. The herbals of the seventeenth century, including Gerarde's, were still quoting Dioscorides and many other classical authorities as the source of their information, though with some quiet revisions and reservations.

RENAISSANCE

As far as medicine was concerned, rediscovered classical ideas led gradually to a questioning of the *status quo*. One of the most important figures of the Florentine Renaissance was Marsilio Ficino (1433–1499), whose patrons were Cosimo, Piero and Lorenzo de Medici. Ficino translated Plato from Greek texts, and the Hermetic Corpus, named after Hermes Trismegistus, which dated in fact to the first century AD, but was thought to have been much older. It contained information about alchemy and other occult matters. Other Renaissance mages such as Cornelius Agrippa added their opinions to the intellectual debate. A kind of philosophical magic entered European thought, influencing not only art, religion and philosophy but medicine as well.

Ficino also wrote an original book with the aim of postponing old age, *Liber de Vita, The Book of Life*. He believed that cosmic forces, the rays of the stars, penetrated the earth, and that gold, silver and precious stones could be used, with the help of astrological images, to cure illness. He had much of interest to say about diet and lifestyle, and the control of the melancholy to which scholars were inclined.[7] It seems likely that this Natural Magic is the rationale behind the use of powdered gems and precious metals in some of the receipts both in the household books and the orthodox medicine of the seventeenth century. Intact precious stones worn for their magical properties had of course been appreciated since classical times.

A serious challenge to Greek and Roman theories came from an iconoclastic Swiss doctor, Paracelsus, the adopted name of Theophrastus Bombastus von Hohenheim, who claimed in this way that he was superior – *para* – to a famous Roman doctor called Celsus. Paracelsus, who died in 1541 at the age of about forty-nine, was an innovator who criticised the Galenic system and introduced some 'chemical' remedies, particularly those based on salt, sulphur and mercury. He was also an alchemist. In a stormy and quarrelsome life, he made many enemies in the medical establishment. At one point, he publicly burned the revered *Canon* of Avicenna while holding an academic position in Basel. His contract was not renewed, so to speak, and he had to leave town hastily.

He spent much time wandering throughout Europe, learning as he went, starting from childhood in the mining schools of the Fugger family, and taking in learning from universities and humble wise-women alike. He stressed that Nature was the teacher, not books, though he wrote extensively himself. His influence on medicine in general was not great during his lifetime, though he was famous for his cures. Gradually, however, some of his ideas gained ground in the next hundred years. One of his receipts for a plaster even found its way into Mrs Corlyon's manuscript: 'The vertues of this Emplaister by Paracelsus ar innumerable.'[8] He thought that distillation cleaned remedies, hence perhaps the overwhelming use of distilled 'waters' in seventeenth-century medicine. In fact, many of the waters are alcoholic, as wines and spirits were frequently used as the vehicle for herbal preparations. He promoted the Doctrine of Signatures, which stated that many herbs had been marked by a benevolent creator with a sign to show what they were good for, a yellow flower for jaundice, for example.

Knowledge of anatomy had made considerable progress in Europe since the Middle Ages. Andreas Vesalius, Professor of Anatomy at the University of Padua, published *De humani corporis fabrica* (On the Structure of the Human Body) in 1543. It was just as useful to artists as to doctors, and was in itself a work of art. Further anatomical work in Padua gave clues to William Harvey about the function of veins. In 1628, he published his discovery of the circulation of the blood. This was a triumph of reasoning, because the capillaries, literally the missing link between arteries and veins, could not be seen until the later development of the microscope. Dissection of the human body remained problematic however, because of religious scruples. There was a shortage of cadavers for medical education. The new knowledge was only slowly accepted, and made very little difference to therapeutic practice. Even eminent physicians were sceptical, let alone the compilers of household remedies.

Culpeper, in the introduction to his translation of the *Pharmacopoeia Londinensis*, carefully explained what he meant by Animal, Vital and Natural spirits. They were three different kinds of power which gave the body sense and motion, life and nourishment.[9] *Animal spirits* were based in the brain. They directed the external senses of sight, hearing and so on, as well as internal senses of imagination, judgment and memory. *Vital spirits* were the source of life, and also positive emotions such as joy and courage, as well as their opposites, sadness, hatred etc. The Vital spirits came from the heart. Lastly the *Natural spirits* nourished the body by altering or concocting food into chyle, chyle into blood, blood into flesh. The word 'concoct' comes from a Latin root meaning to cook, and it was thought that digestion was a kind of cookery carried out in the stomach.

FOLK MEDICINE

Discovering exactly what went on in folk medicine is difficult, because by its nature it was an oral tradition, and as suggested above, secrecy was often wise. However, careful research has revealed a rich list of plants in use from the seventeenth to the nineteenth centuries. Susan Drury's M. Phil. thesis of 1984 gives details of nearly two hundred plants used in folk remedies.[10] David E. Allen and Gabrielle Hatfield, the authors of *Medicinal Plants in Folk Tradition* list even more. The assumption must be that country people used customs, spells, herbs and potions surviving from long ago. Allen and Hatfield point out that in the remoter parts of the countryside, people neither knew nor cared about learned medicine, but relied on local plants.[11] These were most likely effective too, especially for less serious conditions, such as skin diseases, aches and pains. Curiosity and observation were great teachers. It may be thought that anyone who looked after animals, for instance, could notice what plants were eaten by sick beasts, and try them out himself. If something worked, it would become treasured knowledge, to be handed on from granny to grandchild. There was a whole local pharmacopoeia freely available in the fields, woods, hillsides and on the seashore.

The country traditions of the seventeenth century can be thought of, perhaps, as the alternative medicine of the time, and like our own alternative therapies there may well have been some beneficial common-sense input into official wisdom.

The presence of local healers was acknowledged in the so-called 'Quacks' Charter' of 1542, which allowed people with 'knowledge of the nature, kind, and operation of certain herbs, roots and waters' to give 'comfort, succour, help, relief and health [to] the King's poor subjects.'[12] It was a partial reaction to the activities of the College of Physicians of London, which had been formed in 1518. The College had (not unreasonably) sought to license practitioners of medicine in order to raise standards, but this led to bitter demarcation disputes between physicians, apothecaries and barber-surgeons. In any case, there were never enough doctors, and it was impossible to supervise informal treatments. Midwifery, too, was the province of women, either friends, relatives, or women with experience of childbirth licensed by the local bishop. It sounds like a cosy arrangement, but infant and maternal mortality were high by modern standards.

CAUSES OF SICKNESS

What caused disease? Though reverence was paid to Galen, it slowly became obvious that there must be other factors at the root of 'new' afflictions such as syphilis, and epidemics such as plague.

For the religious, sickness of any kind might be a punishment of sin, or like Job's sufferings, a trial of steadfastness. Plague might be thought of as a 'visitation' from God, where the proper course was public prayer, fasting, and repentance.

On the other hand, there might be natural physical causes, as Hippocrates had said. During an epidemic, it was incredible that so many people could suffer the same imbalance of humours at the same time. Some kind of infective agent was at work, spreading the disease, so that quarantine might limit the spread. Going away into the country was an obvious option for the rich. But what was this infective agent? Bad air or smells were blamed by some. A 'miasma' could rise up from filth of any kind, including ditches which were open sewers, uncleaned streets with dead animals, overflowing churchyards, and smelly trades such as tanning leather. It was not difficult to notice a miasma, and be warned. Perfumes were made and used not only aesthetically, but as a health measure. Or perhaps there was some kind of venom in the air (as the Anglo-Saxons thought), in which case you could take a prophylactic such as Venice Treacle to keep the poison out.

Robert Hooke, the great polymath of the early days of The Royal Society, published his *Micrographia* in 1665. He showed a new world revealed by the microscope. He drew a portrait of a flea among many other marvels. Later, the Dutchman, Antony van Leeuwenhoek, using a stronger microscope, discovered 'animalcules'. Only very much later, with the work of Pasteur and Koch, would it be realised that micro-organisms caused infectious diseases.

DISEASES OF THE 17TH CENTURY

Perception of disease has thus changed very much over the past 350 years, and it is impossible to be certain that the ailments described in the past are exactly the same as ours. Where we would think of something like a headache or cough as a symptom of an underlying condition, the seventeenth century housewife turned to her book to find out what to do for 'griefs in the stomach', 'pain in the breast' or swellings in the legs or feet. Some diseases had names, possibly the same names as they have recently been known by – gout, colic, consumption, stone in kidney or bladder for instance. There was ague (a malarial infection), and various fevers. The King's Evil (scrofula) appears. Scurvy is mentioned even in the household books, and there are many eye conditions, such as 'pin and web' and dimness of sight. The notebooks contain a number of treatments for various accidents, such as bruising, burning, wounds, including gunshot, procedures for childbirth, and children's complaints. Mental problems such as lethargy, melancholy and frenzy have their remedies too. Some suggestions are for less serious conditions: baldness, cold in the head, pimples, corns, 'pissing in bed' and the social disadvantage of stinking breath. The manuscripts include recipes for comforting drinks for fevers, and for possets and jellies as invalid food.

Fatal illnesses seen as distinct are listed in the Bills of Mortality. These statistics for London were collected by the Parish Clerks and published weekly, culminating in a Bill for the whole year. The 1665 Bill for London, the year of the Great Plague, gives a total of burials of 97,306. Of these, the terrible number of 68,596 were victims of the plague. This is almost certainly an underestimate.[13]

The Bills were not accurate by our standards. The procedure at the best of times was for a 'searcher' to view the body and determine the cause of death. These searchers were almost always old and illiterate women, with no training but experience, given the job to keep them off poor relief. Their opinions were apt to be unreliable. Still, the range of sickness accorded with the perceptions of the time.

The next biggest killer after the plague in this year was *Ague and Feaver*, with 5,257 fatalities. *Consumption and Tissick*, with nearly 5,000 deaths, came next. *Convulsion and Mother* carried off another 2,036, *Spotted Feaver and Purples* (which may have been a variant of plague), almost 2,000 more. *Teeth and Worms*, came to 2,614. *Teeth* might apply to babes with infections, perhaps attributed to teething. Alternatively, dental caries was thought to be caused by worms in the teeth (see p. 84) so, grouping them together with intestinal parasites, might be logical. (It is a sad thought that one might die of toothache.) *Dropsie and Timpany* accounted for nearly 1,500. *Surfet* killed another 1,251 people, in contrast with *Rickets*, which took 500 or so. *Griping in the Guts* was fairly serious, with 1,288. *Stopping of the Stomach* was comparatively rare, at about 300 cases.

Sadly, *Chrisomes and Infants* had 1,258 deaths. A chrisom child was less than a month old. Mortality among young babies was evidently so commonplace that it was not worth assigning a specific disease to them in the Bills. There were also more than 600 cases of *Abortive and Stillborne*. *Childbed* took 625 women. *Overlaid and Starved* pathetically accounted for 45, though the latter might apply to adults.

Other causes of death, in much smaller numbers, included *Bedrid, Cancer, Gangrene and Fistula, Flox and Smal Pox, Gout and Sciatica, Headmouldshot and Mouldfallen*. There were only four deaths from these last unpleasant afflictions, possibly bone diseases, as a head-mould was another name for a skull. The list continues: *Jaundies, Impostume* (boil or ulcer), *Kings Evill* (scrofula), *Meagrom and Headach, Palsie, Plurisie, Quinsie, Rising of the Lights, Scurvy, Shingles and Swine pox, Stone and Strangury*, and *Vomiting*. *Sores, Ulcers, broken and bruised Limbes* killed eighty-two.

Further violent deaths were included in the statistics. Unfortunates might be *Kild by several accidents*, or more specifically *Blasted, Drowned, Executed, Murthered, and Shot*, or *Poysoned*. A mysterious cause of death, *Plannet* accounted for six fatalities. In later Bills, it is sometimes coupled with *Blasted*, presumably by lightning, so perhaps it was some malign astrological event, or even what we would call a stroke.

What might now be attributed to depression came under the headings of *Distracted, Grief*, and *Hangd & made away with themselves*. The total of these last three causes came to only fifty-eight, not a high proportion I think given the enormous stresses of this year.

All these figures must be put against an estimated population of London of at least 300,000.[14]

3

Herbal Medicine

In the seventeenth-century household books, there are many more herbal cures than those based on animal parts or minerals. The tradition of herbal medicine is vast, stretching from prehistory through all subsequent civilisations. The Egyptians used herbs and unguents not only as medicine, but in the process of embalming their dead. The Greeks produced the great Dioscorides, whose *De materia medica*, written during the first century AD, was the standard pharmacopoeia in the Western and Arab worlds for about fourteen hundred years.

Written herbals had been copied avidly through the Middle Ages and beyond, with Dioscorides' as a basic text. The Anglo-Saxon *Leechbook of Bald* and the *Lacnunga* treatises among others added knowledge of northern European plants to the pot. Several distinguished herbals were available in the seventeenth century. For instance, John Gerarde's *Herball or General Historie of Plantes*, was first published in 1597, and Nicholas Culpeper's *The English Physitian* in 1652. This went through many editions. They were sources of medical receipts and supplementary knowledge, as their purpose was to teach the identification, uses and 'vertues' of plants. Obviously pragmatic knowledge must have been common. Anyone who had to do with herbs would know that senna, for example, was purgative, poppy juice soporific. Shakespeare, for instance, referred to many common English herbs, which suggests that not only he but his audience were familiar with them.

Traditional knowledge and the Galenic system of selecting plants according to their qualities (hot, cold etc.) were not the only criteria

for choosing herbs. Paracelsus' Doctrine of Signatures offered another way. According to this theory, God had mercifully ensured
that something about the plant had an affinity with a particular
disorder or organ. For instance lungwort, with spotted leaves sug-
gesting pulmonary disease, could be used to cure chest complaints.
Plants with yellow flowers, or yellow spices, might be good for
jaundice. This is reflected here and there in the household receipts.
The Barrett manuscript has 'An excelent medicen for the Yallow
jandes & a pain in the Stomack' which contains both saffron and
turmeric mixed with white wine.[1]

It is an interesting fact that some of these herbs do work in the
way they are supposed to, but Gabrielle Hatfield, in *Memory, Wisdom
and Healing*, suggests that the whole system arose from practical
mnemonics.[2] You could easily remember that the lesser celandine
was helpful for piles, for instance, because its root had little nodules
that looked like swellings. (If you named it 'pilewort' that helped
too!)Yet another system was based on astrology. Astrology had
been an accepted part of medical theory in the Middle Ages, but
by early modern times it was on its way out, though still not dis-
credited entirely. Culpeper is an exponent of this system. The book
now called *Culpeper's Herbal* started as *The English Physitian, OR An
Astrologo-Physical Discourse of the Vulgar [common] Herbs of the Nation.*
Each plant was ruled by one of the planets (which included the Sun
and Moon). Every disease and part of the body was also ruled by
one of them, and so a suitable herb could be selected. He saw man
as the microcosm, the small mirror of the mighty macrocosm, an
alchemical and Renaissance concept.

In his address To the Reader he says:[3]

I knew well enough the whole world and everything in it was formed
of a Composition of contrary Elements, and in such a harmony as
must needs shew the wisdom and Power of a great God. I knew
as well this Creation though thus composed of contraries was one
united Body, and man an Epitome of it. I knew those various affec-
tions in man in respect of Sickness and Health were caused Naturally
(though God may have other ends best known to himself) by the
various operations of the *Macrocosm*, and I could not be ignorant, that

as the Cause is, so must the Cure be, and therefore he that would know the reason of the operation of Herbs must look up as high as the Stars; I alwaies found the Disease vary according to the various motion of the stars, and this is enough one would think to teach a man by the Effect where the Cause lay.

In practice, however, the matching of herb to disease was complicated. Herbs might cure either by sympathy (like cures like) or by antipathy (opposites cure). He gave as an example *Carduus Benedictus*, or Blessed Thistle, 'an Herb of *Mars* and under the Sign *Aries*.' By sympathy it could cure giddiness, because the head was governed by Aries, in the house of Mars. It was also good for choleric complaints, red faces and ringworm, and 'helps Plague-sores, Boils and Itch, the Biting of mad Dogs, and venemous Beasts, all which infirmities are under *Mars*.' However, it was also a cure for 'French Pox [syphilis] by Antypathy to *Venus* who governs it. It strengthens the Memory and cures Deafness by Antipathy to *Saturn* ...' (A confused reader could buy and study his other books on astrology.)

How Herbs Work in the Modern View

Some plants are useful in medicine because they contain *alkaloids* which affect the human nervous system. They may be similar in structure to naturally occurring body chemicals. They are frequently poisonous, even deadly in large quantities, so the dosage is critical. Examples are hemlock, henbane and opium, all known for thousands of years and used to relieve pain. Hemlock was the poison administered to Socrates when he was condemned to death.

Many plants contain *essential oils*, familiar today to those people who use them in aromatherapy, as bath scents, or vaporise them to make the house smell sweet. They are complicated in chemical structure, and difficult to synthesise, because many different oils may be present in a single plant. They are said to be *carminative* when they are good for digestion, *expectorant* when they encourage coughing, *stimulant* when they act as a tonic, *diuretic* when they stimulate the production of urine, and *antiseptic* when they help to prevent infection.. The undiluted essential oil of most plants is very strong, and should not be taken internally, or rubbed onto the skin, without dilution.

In most seventeenth-century receipts the essential oils were obtained by soaking the herb in alcohol of some kind, or, for ointments, mixing them with grease such as lard or butter.

Mucilages are slippery carbon compounds. Marsh mallow (the plant) is an example of a frequently used seventeenth century ingredient, often used in cough mixtures. (Snails were seen in the same light.) *Tannins* are astringent, and as the name implies were used for tanning leather. They are frequently contained in the bark of trees, as in the oak for instance.

There are many other actions of plants as well. They may be laxative, emetic, emollient, bitter, rubefacient (making the skin warm and red), and so on. Some are vulnerary, helping to heal wounds, or anthelmintic, to destroy intestinal worms. Anti-lithic herbs were especially prized, as stones in kidney or bladder were common in the seventeenth century. In short, there is/was a herb thought to cure or relieve most ills, although in practice they may not have worked as well as the receipts claim.

All these are modern explanations, however, based on scientific analyses. As we have seen, the seventeenth-century rationale sometimes differed from ours. Firstly, as we should think reasonable, a plant was used because long tradition suggested that *X* herb was good for *Y* condition, but at other times, it was used because it re-balanced humours, or had God's signature upon it, or was astrologically desirable. Thus, according to Gerarde, 'Wilde Time boiled in wine and drunke, is good against the wambling and gripings of the bellie ...' and it 'is hot and drie in the third degree: it is of thinn and subtill partes, cutting and much biting'.[4] Culpeper agrees that the oil is 'very heating'. It was a plant of Venus, and among other uses, an infusion was 'a certain remedy for that troublesome complaint, the night-mare.'[5]

SIMPLES

Simples were plants used alone. The term could also be used to describe herbs as gathered. They were typically the ones that grew wild (and free) in a particular locality. They were the root and branch of old wives' remedies, but were also the basis of physicians' medicines and apothecaries' stock-in-trade. The idea of an active principle in any particular plant seems to have been proposed by Paracelsus, but the proof came much later with modern chemistry.

Some remedies, simple in both senses, draw on this traditional knowledge. They would probably have been effective. For example:

> for the Collick or wind in the body [6]
> Take a pint of muscadine and 6 or 7 spoonfulls of the Juice of sage, and mingle them togather and take 2 or 3 spoon fulls euery morning.

Sage is good for dyspepsia – hence its traditional use in stuffing with rich meats, as an aid to digestion:

> A Medecine to stanch Bleedinge at the Nose [7]
> Take Isope and bruse it, then putt it in a clothe and holde it to your Nose and it will stopp it.

Bruised green hyssop, applied to cuts, is said to heal them quickly:[8]

> For a Burne, or a Scalde [9]
> Take a raw onyon, chop it very small, or beat it in a mortar, bruise it with a knife or spoon, & put it between Cambrick or Tiffanie unstarch'd and applie it to the part greiued. If there remaynes anie rednesse, put more of the same to it, & it will take it away.
> This doth good, although used a day or two after ./.
> Mris. Gregorie

Onion-juice for burns has a pedigree elevated from folk-medicine. Gerarde says:

The juice taketh away the heat of scalding with water or oile, as also burning with fire & gunpouder, as is set forth by a very skilfull Surgeon Mr William Clowes one of the Queens Surgeon; and before him by Ambrose Parey, in his treatise of wounds made by gun-shot. [10]

Ambroise Paré was the great French surgeon of the sixteenth century, who pioneered more humane and effective methods of treating battle-wounds We now know that onions have antibiotic properties, so they would help to prevent infection of the damaged tissues. They were still being used thus in East Anglia in modern times. [11] (In the past they were also thought to attract infection into themselves, like disease- magnets, to keep a person carrying them, or a whole household, safe from contagion.)

Extracting Virtues

The herbs could be used alone, as in the above remedies, just by mashing them up, or sometimes by mashing them and then pressing out the juice. However, most internal medicines, ointments and so on were made from several plants and other ingredients. Some of them were of great complexity, as described later. To extract the virtue or curative substance there were many different ways of treating the herbs.

Infusing in a liquid was straightforward. Anyone who has recently made a cup of tea has carried out the process. The herbs might be dried or fresh. Cold infusions were done when the herb was delicate and heat would have spoilt it. A compromise was possible, with just-warm liquid. The following receipt explains the method in detail, and is also a good example of a plain syrup. It is by Gideon Harvey, a doctor who was concerned to help his patients keep their money out of the pockets of the apothecaries:

The Description of Syrupus Garyophyllorum, or Syrup of Gillyflowers. [12]
Take fragrant Gilliflowers, cut off from their white strings, one pound; pour on them a quart of Spring Water, and let them stand

all night. Then strain the Liquor, and being gently warmed, dissolve therein four pound of the whitest Sugar, without boiling it.

The Manner of preparing.

1. Buy the most fragrant Gilliflowers, that are newly gathered, at ten or twelve pence the peck.

2. Put them into a large pewter Flagon, or a new earthen glased Pipkin, and pour the Water, being warmed, upon them; then stop your Flagon, or earthen Veszel very close, and place it all night in the Cellar.

3. Strain off your tinctured liquor, without much pressing the Strainer, in regard you are not to clarifie it, as other Liquors are for Syrups; for that would occasion a great loss of those fragrant Cordial Spirits.

4. Place your Syrup-pan over a very gentle charcoal fire burning clear without the least smoak, and let your liquor be only luke-warm; then put in the Sugar, being powdered and sifted gradually, stirring it about very gently with a long Steel Spatula, or slice (which you may buy big enough for your turn for ten pence at the Rasor-makers) as soon as you find the Sugar all dissolved, take it off immediately, without letting it boil or be hot.

Decoctions were prepared when the ingredient was tough, and when simply soaking in hot water would not do. It had to be boiled to extract the goodness. Roots often came into this category, or hard seed-heads, as here:

Syrup of Poppies, the lesser Composition [13]
Take the heads of white Poppies and black, when both of them are green [unripe], of each six ounces; the seeds of Lettice, of the flowers of Violets, of each one ounce, boyl them in eight pints of Water, till the vertue is out of the heads, then strain them, and with four pound of Sugar boyl the Liquor to a syrup.

This was one of several receipts for soporific syrups. Care was needed with all of them. 'I desire they may be used with a great deal of caution and wariness ... not fit to be given in the beginnings of Feavers, nor to such whose bodies are costive'.

Tinctures are similar to infusions or decoctions, but the liquid used contains alcohol. Occasionally in the household receipts stronger alcohol was used, but most commonly ale or wine was the liquid of choice. Heating would reduce the alcoholic content of the mixture, leaving the 'vertue' in the remaining liquid.

Distillates. There was a passion for distilling medicines. The actual process is comparatively easy. A mushy substance such as pounded herbs, or a liquid, is heated until a vapour is formed, and this vapour is then cooled so that it condenses back into liquid. (Everyone today must have noticed that when vegetables are simmered in a covered saucepan the lid drips when you remove it from the pan.) Exactly what is extracted from the original substance depends on its composition and the degree of heat applied. Alcohol, for example, has a lower boiling point than water, so that a gentle heat will drive off the alcohol first. Many receipts specify that you should keep the 'first water' separate from the rest. Very many 'waters' have an alcoholic component.

In practice, special equipment is needed. Alchemists had long practice in this during the Middle Ages, and developed various kinds of stills, or alembics as they were sometimes called, though an alembic was strictly the top part of the apparatus. Some were made of metal, some of glass or pottery. A person poured the starting herbs, flowers etc., or liquid, into the body of the container, then covered it with a closely fitting head, using dough or sticky paper to seal the join. At the top or side of the head was a long open spout, often curved. The still was then heated, frequently by putting it in a bed of warm ashes or sand. Sometimes, the air in the room was cool enough to condense the vapour in the spout, so that it dripped into a receiving glass or pot, sometimes other measures such as an enclosing water-bath or wet rags round the spout were used to cool it down.

Here is Gideon Harvey explaining to the frugal householder how he could produce a simple herb-water from fresh herbs, much more cheaply than he could buy it:

The manner of distilling the said Simple Waters[14]
Put as many of those Herbs [such as balm or red poppy flowers] (being separated from the greater stalks) or Flowers (pull'd from their husks) as will only fill two Thirds, or at most three Fourth parts of the body of a Pewter Alembick, or a Copper Alembick with a Bucket head,

without adding any Water to the Herbs (which too many *Apothecaries* do) and having closed the head to the body, by pasting slips of Paper of the breadth of an inch, or a little more, round about the juncture, with Starch or Yest; kindle your fire gradually, and continue it to a heat so gentle, that your hand may endure it on any part of the Head; and so you will distill your Waters without smelling of being burn'd, provided you have put ashes to the thickness of an inch and half between the plate and the body or bottom of your Pewter Alembick.

If you make use of a Copper Alembick, you must fill the bucket with cold Water, and as soon as you find the Water to be hot in the said bucket head, you must tap it off, and fill it up again with cold Water.

The reason you are not to fill the body of the Alembick with Herbs, is, because should you fill it up, the bottom of the cake of the Herbs will be dried and burn'd before the top is half dry or distilled off.

Such simple distillation was thought to be a method of purifying and concentrating the virtue of the plant.

CORDIALS

Originally, a cordial was something good for the heart, a tonic for the vital spirits upon which life itself depended. The word itself comes from the Latin *cor, cordis*, heart. Cordials were pleasant to drink, with a convivial air about them. The word 'cordial' has survived, now meaning warm and friendly, or, as a noun, often implying a concentrated soft drink, of lime juice, for example. Seventeenth-century cordials are usually based on fruit, plus alcohol, and sometimes, but not always, distilled again.

This one is by H. S. who contributed to the Barrett manuscript:

A Cordiall Water of S[i]r Water Rayleys [15]
Take a gallon of straberies & put into them a pint of aquavita let them stand so 4. or 5. dayes, then straine them out gently & sweeten the water with fine sugar.

Another from *The Queen's Closet* is very much like a modern cherry-brandy, though we would use more cherries to the brandy, even with a smaller seventeenth-century liquid measure:

A Cordial Cherry-water.[16]
Take a pottle of Aqua vitae [half a gallon], two ounces of ripe Cherries stoned, Sugar one pound, twenty four Cloves, one stick of Cinnamon, three spoonfuls of aniseeds bruised, let these stand in the Aqua vitae fifteen days, and when the water hath fully drawn out the tincture, pour it off into another glass for your use, which keep close stopped, the Spice and the Cherries you may keep, for they are very good for winde in the Stomach.

POLYPHARMACY

However, a large number of remedies in the household books are much more complicated than the above receipts. Very many different herbs, spices and sometimes chemicals are treated in various ways. They are pounded in a mortar, macerated, strained, distilled, left in the sun or buried in the ground or in an ant-hill – presumably to maintain an even temperature.

Why were so many different ingredients called for? We know today that a mixture of several substances may work synergistically, being more effective than the sum of its parts. Or because there were many reasons for choosing a plant, any one herb might be used to help a number of different symptoms. This may partly explain why some compound medicines were used for a huge range of illnesses in a way which seems alien if not ridiculous today.

Or, perhaps a range of herbs was suggested so that whatever was obtainable could be used, and it wouldn't matter if one or two were left out. Or, if one herb didn't work, another might. The suspicion grows though that one ingredient may cancel out another. The seventeenth-century rationale might have been that because one herb was good for you, a whole gardenful must be that much better.

PANACEAS

Galen's medicine was what we would now call holistic. When one was ill, the whole person was perceived to be sick. It followed then that an effective medicine which treated the entire body might restore health, even though several different organs were affected. The same rationale applied to the Elixir of the alchemists, of course, which, in theory, would make the body as perfect as it could become.

In practice, very elaborate medicines were prepared. They were venerable receipts, having been developed from classical authorities, such as Galen himself, Avicenna, Dioscorides and many others. Gerarde is especially scrupulous in naming his authorities and so is Culpeper, but the general run of writers were less inclined to cite their sources, though there are notable exceptions to this. More or less contemporary physicians are often credited. A Dr Stevens and a Dr Butler are frequently mentioned for instance.

Several multi-purpose cures appear over and over again. The popular *Aquamirabilis* (wonderful water) is sometimes given more than once in the same manuscript. (Kidder has two.) It appears early and late in the century. Here is Mrs Corlyon's version in 1606 with not only *mirabilis* but with *pretiosa* (precious) as well:

The makinge and vertues of Aqua mirabilis et pretiosa [17]
Take Gallingale Cloues Cubibes Gynger Melylott Cardimony Maces Nuttmegges of eche a dramm made into powder, and mingle all these powders togeather, with halfe a pinte of the iuyce of Selendine, a pinte of good Aquauite and three pintes of good white wine. Putt all these togeather in a Stillytory of glasse, and lett it stand so all nighte and in the morninge distyll it with as easye a fyer as may be. This water is of secreat and excellent vertue. Viz It dissolueth the swellinge of the Lunges without any greefe, and if the Lunges be perished or wounded, it much helpeth and comforteth them. It preserueth the Bloode from putrefaction and he shall neuer neede to be lett Bloode that vseth this water. It suffereth not the Harte to be brent, nor Melancholye or Fleame to be lifte vpp or haue dominion aboue Nature.

It expellethe the Rhewme, profyteth the Stomake and conseru-
ethe the Bodye in very good estate. It engendrethe coulour, and
keepeth and conserueth the visage and memorye. It is good for the
winde Collicke and it destroyeth the Palsye of Lymmes and tounge.
A spoonefull of this water geuen to a man or woeman laboringe
towardes Deathe releeueth [relieveth]. Of all waters arteficiall this
is the best. In the Sommer use thereof fastinge, once a weeke to
the quantitye of a spoonefull and in the winter two spoonefulles
likewise fastinge.

This is truly a wide-spectrum remedy. The lungs are taken care
of, and the sanguine humour, blood, kept in good condition without a plethora, which would otherwise call for blood-letting. The
heart will be undamaged, and melancholy and phlegmatic humours
maintained in correct proportions. It dries up rheums, or runny
noses and eyes, is good for the stomach and therefore digestion,
as well as dealing with colic. It is a general tonic, giving a healthy
colour, and keeping face and memory in good fettle – young, in
other words, additionally curing shakiness of the limbs and disorder
of the tongue. It won't hold off death forever, but will ease the
passage of those whose time has come.

A receipt from the end of the century [18] has the same basic
ingredients plus several more. Now included are a dram each of
elecampane and orange peel, a half pint each of spearmint and balm
juice and double the amount of celandine juice. There are additionally handfuls of rosemary, borage, violet and half a handful
of marigold flowers. As these are fresh flowers, 'the onely time for
makeing it is in may.' The mixture is allowed to stand for two days
before distilling, and the distillate is separated into three lots. It is
said to be of 'rare virtue' but the diseases are unspecified. Possibly
it didn't seem quite so wonderful by this time.

'Dr Stevens' Water' is another such, making many appearances
in different collections, including Sir Hugh Plat's. [19] Here is the
version from the Barrett manuscript, with a testimonial from the
Archbishop of Canterbury attached:

Dr Steevens Water given by himself to the arch Bishop of Canterbury[20]
Take a gallon of gascon wine, then take ginger, gallingall, cinamon,
nutmeges, cloves, graines, aniseeds, fenell seeds of every one of them
a dram, then take caraway seeds of red mints, roses, time, camamile
the leaves if you cannot come by the flowers, & pellitorie of the
Wale, rose-mary wild time of Small Lavender of each a handfull,
then break the spices small, & shread the hearbs & put all into the
Wine & let it stand 12 hours stirring it divers times in a day, then still
it in a limbeck, & keep the first water, & the second water is good
but not so good as the first. If it be set in the Sun all the sumer it
will be the better

The Vertue of this Water
It comforteth the vital Spirrits, & helps all inward diseases that come
of cold. it is good against the shaking of the palsie, it cures the con-
traction of the sinews, it helpeth the conception of a Woman, if they
be barren, it kills the worms in the belly & Stomach, it cures the cold
dropsie, & helpeth the Stone in the Blader, or in the reines [kidneys]
of the back, it helpeth a stinking breath. Who so ever useth this water
morning & eving [sic] it will make him look young & comforteth
nature marvelousley./.

With this water Dr Stevens preserved his life till he co[u]ld neither
goe nor stand with extreem old age, & said this was all the medison
he took in his sickness at any time.
The Arch Bishop used it at any time when he was sick, & at some
other times to comfort him, & he lived to a great age.

The same did Mr Law-worth, & at his death recomended it to all men.

Mr Law-worth's recommendation of the 'water' on his death-bed
strikes me as slightly ironic, though at this time death was set apart
from illness. One's death was in the hands of God, whereas sickness
was amenable to human cure.

The *Treasvrie of Hidden Secrets* gives details of the transmission
of the receipt to a grateful public. I quote the title from this book
in full:

How to make a soveraigne water, that M. Doctor Stephens, Physician, a man of great knowledge and cunning [skill] did practice, and used of long experience, and therewith did very many cures, and kept it alwaies secret, till of late a little before his death, Doctor Parker, late Archbishop of Canterbury, did get it in writing of him.[21]

Matthew Parker, 1504–1575 was an Elizabethan Archbishop. He had also been the fourteenth Master of Corpus Christi College, Cambridge, between 1544–1553. A discriminating collector of manuscripts and early printed works, he left his books to the College, where they still remain as the Parker Library. He (or perhaps his wife, Margaret) was evidently interested in practical knowledge as well as academic subjects. He was known to take an interest in gardening, and a small cookery book has been found among other texts belonging to him.[22] His success in preserving a secret receipt for a cordial water is in character. His 'great age' when he died was seventy-one. According to the *Treasvrie*, this water also 'preserved Doctor Stevens, that he lived fourscore and eighteen yeares [ninety-eight], whereof ten yeares he lived bedred.'

Extravagant claims of this kind probably did increase confidence in taking such general tonics. The separation of distilled medicines into first and second waters appears elsewhere. The first water would have contained the more volatile substances, which would have evaporated first, as explained above. The second water contained the ones more difficult to vaporise. Perhaps a slight aura of alchemy clings to the whole proceeding, especially as the medicine is credited with bringing about an appearance of youth. One of the aims of alchemy was to find a means of staying young and achieving a very long life, if not immortality.

'Lucastala's Balsame' is another all-purpose remedy, based on Venice turpentine washed in water and rose water, with wax, olive oil, and red sanders.[23] It was a salve for wounds, burns, ulcers and fistulas, worms and cancers, aches, headache, and indigestion, colic and not least, piles (applied externally). Taken internally it was good for poison or surfeit, smallpox and measles, and the bites of venomous snakes and scorpions. Smeared on lips and nostrils it prevented infection.

Isaac Newton was said to treat himself with 'Lacatellus Balsam' if he thought he might be developing consumption. He would take about a quarter of a pint at a time internally. He also applied it externally for wounds.[24]

Venice turpentine is the resin of the European larch. In this form it would have been a solid, not a modern paint-thinner. It is a disinfectant, and Pepys mentions taking it. On 31 December, 1664, he remarks that he is in good health, despite the cold weather. 'But I am at a great losse to know whether it be my hare's foote [an amulet against colic], or taking every morning of a pill of turpentine, or my having left off the wearing of a gowne.'[25] (He wore a coat instead.)

As one of the uses of the Lucastella's balsam was to counteract the stinging of scorpions, not often encountered in Britain, it is likely that the preparation originated abroad. I haven't been able to trace Lucastella, or his variants elsewhere of Lucattella, Lucantella, but his name has a classical air about it. The Barrett receipt adds a note about him:

> Lucastela the authour, to give the better satisfaction of the goodness & worth of the said balsom, cured himself being with scalded lead scalded and greace of pork [i.e. being scalded with hot lead and pork fat] & having pierced his side in the presence of diverse persons healed it agayne, to the admiration & astonishment of them all.

It would be interesting to know when the demonstration took place and who the 'diverse persons' were – friends of friends, perhaps.

MITHRIDATE AND TREACLE

Mithridate features in many cures. It was one of the great standbys of seventeenth-century medicine – indeed for years before that, too. It gets its name from King Mithradates, a king of Pontus in northern Anatolia, who died in 63 BC. After a brutal but at first fairly successful life spent in conquest, he was at last defeated by Pompey. His son turned against him, and he tried to commit suicide by poison, but when this didn't work he ordered a soldier to kill him instead. The failure to die by poison seems to have given rise to the legend that no poison could kill him, and hence he must have taken antidotes against all poisons during his lifetime. The idea of a universal antidote was probably especially attractive to powerful men with ruthless enemies. Among Gerarde's entries for rue,[26] he gives his own translation of a poem by the Latin poet Macer, who died *c*. 47 BC:

> Rue drunke with wine, or eaten rawe,
> withstandeth poysons strong;
> This *Mithridates* king of Pont
> tride oft and prooued long ...

According to the poem, the king ate a score of rue leaves with salt when he first got up in the morning, and felt himself safe from any poison.

Other sources suggest much more complicated concoctions. Culpeper gives a receipt containing fifty herbal ingredients, as well as wine and honey. He attributes his recipe to Democrates, but says 'I have not time to search whether there by any difference in the Composition between *Democrates* and the Colledg [of Physitians] ... but because the Electuary is very chargeable [expensive] to be made and cannot be made but in great quantities, ... I am willing to spare my pains in any further search.' By implication, this was not something to be lightly undertaken at home, but bought as needed from the apothecary or druggist.[27] It was a remarkable medicine, however. Culpeper adds his own comment to the receipt, which he had translated from the London Physicians' *Dispensatory*:

> It is good against poyson, and such as have done themselves wrong by taking filthy medicines, it provokes sweat, it helps continual watrings of the stomach, ulcers in the body, consumptions, weakness of the limbs, rids the body of cold humors, and diseases coming of cold, it remedies cold infirmities of the brain, and stopping of the passage of the sences (viz. hearing, seeing, smelling &c.) by cold, it expels wind, helps the Chollick, provokes appetite to ones victuals, it helps ulcers in the bladder if Galen say true, as also difficulty of urine, it casts out

the dead child, and helps such women as cannot conceive by reason of cold, it is an admirable remedy for melancholly and all diseases of the body coming through cold, it would fill a whol sheet of paper to reckon them all up particularly. You may take a scruple or half a drachm in the morning and follow your business, two drachms will make you sweat, yea one drachm if your body be weak, for then two drachms may be dangerous because of its heat ... [28]

Venice Treacle was another elaborate preparation. It was an electuary (a powder mixed with syrup) developed in Italy. The mixture of drugs and spices was a Roman antidote against poison. In seventeenth-century London it was usually bought from the apothecary but again Culpeper explains how it is made according to the London Physicians. He heads the receipt 'Andromachus *his Treacle*', with a marginal note '*This is that which commonly is called* Venice Treacle'. So that you can judge the amount of effort and skill that went into procuring the ingredients and manufacturing the medicine, I give it almost in full:

Take of Troches of Squils eight and fourty drachms; Troches of Vipers, Long Pepper, Opium of Thebes. Magma Hedycroi, of each 24. drachms; dried Rose leaves, [marginal note Take it alwaies for red Roses, when the other are not mentioned] the whites being cut off, Illyrick Orris, juyce of Liquoris, the seeds of sweet Navew, Scordium, Opobalsamum, Cinnamon, Agrick, of each twelve drachms; Mirrh, sweet Costos, or Zedoary, Saffron, Cassia Ligna, Indian Spicknard, Schoenanth, Pepper white and black, male Frankinsence [margin Olibanum] Dittany of Creet, Rhubarb, Stoechas, Horehound, the seeds of Macedonian Parsly, dried Calaminth, Turpentine, the roots of Cinkfoyl and Ginger, of each six drachms: the branches of Polly-mountain, Camaepitys, Celtick Spicknard, Amomus, Styrax Calamitis, the roots of Spignel, the tops of Germander, the roots of Rhapontick, earth of Lemnos, Indian Leaf, Chalcitis, or instead thereof Roman Vitriol, burnt Gentian roots, Gum Arabick, juyce of Hypocistis, Carpobalsamum or Nutmegs or Cubebs, the seeds of Annis, Fennel, Seseli, or Heartwort, Cardamoms, Acacia, or in lieu thereof the juyce of Sloes made thick, the seeds of Treacle Mustard, the tops of St Johns wort, the seeds of Bishops weed, Sagapenum, of each four drachms: Castorium, the roots of long Birthwort, Bitumen Judaicum, the seeds of Carrots, Opopanax, Centaury the less, Galbanum, of each two drachms: old Canary wine sufficient to dissolve the things that can be dissolved, pure Honey three times the weight of the dry Simples: mix them together according to art.

The vertues of it are, It resists poyson and the bitings of venemous beasts, inveterate headaches, vertigo, deafness, the falling sickness, astonishment, apoplexies, dulness of sight, want of voice, asthmaes, old and new coughs, such as spit or vomit blood, such as can hardly spit or breath, coldness of the stomach, wind, the chollick, the Illiack passion, the yellow jaundice, hardness of the spleen, stone in the reins and bladder, difficulty of urine, ulcers in the bladder, feavers, dropsies, leprosies; it provokes the terms, brings forth both birth and afterbirth, helps pains in the joynts, it helps not only the body, but also the mind, As vain fears, melancholly &c. and is a good remedy in pestilential feavers. Thus Galen. You may take half a drachm and go about your business, and it will do you good if you have occasion to go in ill airs, or in pestilential times; if you shall sweat upon it, as your best way is, if your body be not in health, then take one drachm, or between one and two, or less than one, according as age or strength is; if you cannot take this or any other sweating medicine by it self, mix it with a little Carduus or Dragons water, or Angelica water which in my opinion is the best of the three.[29]

Troches of vipers is an interesting ingredient, linking this receipt with *theriac*, often synonymous with treacle in these receipts. Troches of vipers were made of the flesh of the reptiles boiled with dill, salt and white breadcrumbs, then pressed into little cakes. A refinement was to mark them with the image of a snake.[30] *Theriac*, *theriacal* comes from a Greek root, meaning to pertain to wild beasts and venomous serpents. There was a very old belief that because vipers were immune to their own poison, their flesh was an antidote to their bites. *Treacle* comes from the same root. In the seventeenth century medical sense, it had nothing to do with molasses, which we now call (black) treacle.

There seemed to be an assumption that all poisons were much alike, so could be treated by a universal medicine – hence all the 'bites of venemous beasts' in general. But the plague or pestilence seems also to have been regarded as a kind of poisoning at times – probably from a maisma or poisoned air. Hence theriac or treacle was also used especially as a precaution against getting plague in the first place.

As you can see, Venice Treacle was expensive, so there was a variant, London Treacle, made of hartshorn, native herbs, opium, and easily obtained spices, plus Canary wine and honey. It was still useful, though cheaper: '… a pretty cordial, resists the pestilence, and is a good antidote in pestilential times, it resists poyson, strengthens cold stomachs, helps digestion and crudities of the stomach …'[31]

These complicated compounds belong to a culture which is very far from the oral country tradition of simples. They may, or may not, have been curative, but the patient would have the satisfaction of knowing that a great deal of time, effort and expense went into making the medicine, and that in itself would have been comforting.

4

Accidents and Emergencies

One of Culpeper's receipts in the *Physical Directory*, translated from Latin, was 'A drink for wounded men':[1]

> And therefore lest my poor wounded Country man should perish for want of an *Angel* to Fee a Physitian, or if he have it, before the Physitian (which in some places is very remote) can come at him: I have taken the pains to write the Receipt in his own Mother tongue; he may get any friend to make it...

He adds an acerbic marginal joke, referring to the Bible story: '*Too many Physitians in England being like* Balaams *Asse, they will not speak unless they see an Angel: yet I accuse not all.*' An angel was a coin, as well as a heavenly spirit.

This was part of his campaign against the College of Physicians, yet is a justified statement about the peril of having accidents if you lived in the country – and accidents could happen to anyone. People rode horses, used carts, farmed the land with ploughs and hand-tools. Any careless moment could bring disaster. You could tread on an adder, or a rusty nail. Inquisitive children could eat poisonous berries. Many bees for honey meant many stings. There might be a mad dog in the undergrowth, or an angry pig ready to nip someone's leg. In winter there was ice to slip on. At home, there were risks from candles and rush-lights, open fires in the kitchen, and ladders to climb. All trades had their hazards.

Suppose you fell and broke your leg. There was of course no ambulance to a local hospital for emergencies. Perhaps the doctor's angel was beyond your means, and anyway you couldn't wait for him. Your neighbours and family had better be good at first aid.

It would have been reassuring for them to be able to consult the kitchen notes on physic, or a printed book which included treatments for wounds as well as diseases. In practice, the external treatments were probably more useful than some of the internal medicines. Unlike fevers, nobody could argue about the cause of injury, and therefore about the treatment of something as obvious as falling off a horse. The practical experience of many hundreds of years would have been handed down by country people in the treatment of broken bones, sprains, bruises, scalds and so on.

Pain Relief

Very ancient too was knowledge of herbs that could ease pain. White (opium) poppy, hemlock, henbane and mandrake were well established medicines by Anglo-Saxon times,[2] and continued to be used throughout the Middle Ages. For example, there was an anaesthetic containing hemlock juice given before surgery: 'for to maken a drynke that men calle dwale, to make a man slep-en whyles men karue hym [while men cut him].'[3] This dwale also contained pig's gall (that of a spayed sow for a woman), juice of briony, lettuce, poppy and henbane. To bring the person round, one washed his temples and cheeks with salt and vinegar.

A medieval Augustinian hospice flourished at Soutra Aisle, south-east of Edinburgh, from the twelfth to the fifteenth centuries, and is now the subject of archaeo-medical investigation, careful forensic tests being carried out especially on the contents of the drains that once served the hospital. Once the seeds of the herbal plants had been used to make medicine they were discarded, and, being found in association with other medical waste, prove that such plant material was really used at this time, confirming the written evidence. Pollen analysis shows that flax, hemp and opium poppy were cultivated at the site.[4]

Narcotics are dangerous. Gerarde warns against the use of opium 'the condensed juice of Poppy heads', which although taken internally or applied externally to the head caused sleep, 'somewhat too plentifully taken doth also bring death.'[5] Yet severe pain was dangerous in itself. Culpeper translates a receipt which, he makes clear, is useful in agony as a temporary palliative. He recognises too that pain itself can 'bring a feaver', and cause death, though we might attribute the death to shock in cases of injury:

Philonium Romanum [6]

Take of white Pepper, the seeds of white Henbane, of each five drams; Opium two drachms and an half; Cassia Lignea one drachm and an half; the seeds of Smallage one drachm; the seeds of Macedonian Parsly, Fennel, and Carrots of *Creet*, of each two scruples and five grains; Saffron a scruple and an half; Indian Spicknard, Pellitory of Spain, Zedoary, of each fifteen grains; Cinnamon a drachm and an half; Euphorbium, Mirrh, Castorium, of each one drachm: with three times the weight of them all in clarified Honey, make them into an Electuary according to art.

It is a most exquisite thing to ease vehement and deadly pains, in what part of the body soever they be, whether internal or external; that vehemency of pain will bring a feaver, and a feaver death, no man well in his wits will deny; therfore in such diseases which cause vehemency of pain, as Chollicks, the Stone, Strangury &c. this may be given (ordered by the discretion of an able brain, for it conduceth little to the cure) to mitigate the extremity of pain, until convenient remedy may be had: (as men pump water out before they can stop the hole of a leaking vessel.) …

Mandrake, which had had a sinister reputation in the Middle Ages, was still a herb to induce sleep and reduce anguish, but Gerarde denied many of the legends associated with it. It had been said to grew naturally only under a gallows. It had to be pulled up by a dog (perhaps expendable), which had been tied to it, because it screamed as it was uprooted, causing death to any person who heard it. 'All which dreames and old wives tales you

shall from henceforth cast out of your bookes and memory ...
for I my selfe and my servants also have digged up, planted, and
replanted very many.'[7] At last some hearsay was being challenged
by experience.

BROKEN BONES

Gervase Markham had good advice if a broken bone needed to be
set. His plaster was made with flour and egg whites, both easily
available from the kitchen when needed. The paste becomes firm
and hard on drying:

> A soueraigne help for broken bones.[8]
> Make a plaister of wheat flower and the whits of egges, and spread it
> on a double linnen cloth, and lay the plaister on an euen boord, and
> lay the broken limbe thereon, and set it euen according to nature,
> and lap the plaister about it and splint it, and giue him to drink
> *Knitwort* [probably comfrey], the iuyce thereof, twice and no more,
> for the third time it will vnknit, but giue him to drinke nine dayes
> each day twice the iuyce of *comfrey*, *daisies*, and *osmund* [a fern] in stale
> Ale and it shal knit it, and let the fore-said playster lye to [remain],
> ten dayes at the least ...

Comfrey, also known as knit-bone, may cause healing to take
place too fast, with excess of bone. Here it is given diluted after
the second strong dose. It had been known to help the healing of
broken bones for thousands of years, and it is still valued in modern
herbal medicine.

Anyone who has suffered from uncomfortable plaster will be
glad to know that after ten days the splints were removed, the plaster
soaked with a herbal infusion until it could be removed easily, the
limb cherished with ointment and the process continued with fresh
plaster and splints. There is even a physiotherapy hint: 'if the hurt
be on his arme let him beare a bal of greene hearbs in his hand to
preuent the shrinking of the hand and sinewes.' Nowadays a tennis
ball takes the place of the herbs to exercise the hand.

'Plaster' was not only used for broken bones. The term referred
to many kinds of stiff dressings for wounds, or a means of applying
curative ingredients to the skin. 'A Plaister of Betony'[9] claimed to
do more than immobilise the broken bits. 'It is a gallant Plaister
to unite the skul when it is cracked, to draw out pieces of broken
bones and cover the bones with flesh; It draws filth from the bottom
of deep ulcers, restores flesh lost, clenseth, digesteth and drieth.' It
was made from green betony, burnet, agrimony, sage, pennyroyal,
yarrow, comfrey the greater, clary, frankinsence, mastic, orris, and
round birthwort. The herbs were boiled in wine, strained, and the
mixture stiffened with white wax and several tree gums, including
Venice turpentine, which was antiseptic.

Betony and agrimony were used by Markham 'To draw out bones
broken in the head'.[10] Agrimony, which is still said to be good for
head injury, was crushed and applied to the wound, while betony
juice was given to drink. This herb had a long tradition as a cure
for headaches especially.

ACHES, SPRAINS AND BRUISES, WOUNDS IN GENERAL

Receipts to relieve bruises and sprains are common in all the printed
and manuscript collections. They may be elaborate or plain. In
polypharmacy, a prized remedy was (hopefully) good for many
different conditions. Specific remedies for specific complaints are
the result of experience rather than learned theory.

Mrs Corlyon has a number of 'oyntements' and oil rubs. This
one uses St John's wort, which had the added advantage in folklore
of getting rid of evil spirits:

An Oyntement of St Johns woorte good for all Aches, and is good
eyther of itselfe or to be putt in Salues for watering Soores. It is also
good for any Pricke or greene Wounde [11]
Take of St Johns woorte a weeke before Midsommer or a weeke
after stripe it from the Stalkes, choppe it smale, stampe it with freshe
Hogges grease temper it like doughe and putt it into an earthen pott
and so lett it stand and rott the space of a fortenighte or 3 weekes

Then boile it vppon a soft fyer the space of an hower and after straine
it and so putt it vpp into a Vessell and keepe it for your vse.

Here is another plain remedy supplied by a Mrs Green to Mrs
Miller's book:

An Excellent receipt for a Sprain [12]
Take a Quart of the Lees of wine or the same Quantity of the Grouns
of Strong Beer; Put into it a good handfull of wormwood the same
Quantity of Ground Ivy, and Chickenweed, and marshmallows;
Boyle these all well together, and lay the herbs as hott as you can to
the place, and repeat it 3 or 4 times binding the herbs on If you have
any dear [deer] Suet Stir in a Little Mrs Greens

This combined the virtues of the herbs applied to the skin with the
comfort of a hot poultice. The chickweed and marsh mallow might
have helped to sooth the sore skin. Binding the herbs on would have
helped too, by bandaging the affected part.

Miss Moor's remedy was more problematic, though Kidder records it with approval – *probatum* – at the end:

How to make mis moors oyntm[en]t for a bruise or a Crushe [13]
Take of bay leaues elder leaues Isope Camomill Sothernwood wormwood lauender of each 2 handfulls then take 4lb of unwashed butter
a pottle of blacke snayles [? slugs], boyle them altogather then take
an once of the whitest frankincense and 9 or 10 of the whitest henn
Dungs you can find and when it is almost boyld enough then put in
the 2 last mentioned things and lett it boyle a little more than strayne
itt and keepe itt for your use probatum

Nowadays, the addition of any kind of dung to a medicament seems
totally inappropriate. However, it was an ingredient in many different therapies of the seventeenth century, and I shall return to the
reasons for this later (see p. 191).

Slugs and snails slide into many receipts, for external and internal
use. (See p. 104 for their use in consumption.) Mrs Corlyon has an
elaborate 'golden Oyle good for all Aches and Bruses', which she

attributes to a Mr Burghen.[14] One handful each of thirty different herbs were bruised, put into a glass container with best olive oil and left in the sun for a month. After boiling it up a quart of white wine was added and boiled until the wine had evaporated. The resulting oil was cooled, strained and stored. She adds a note to this:

> Black Snayles also gathered in Maye and put in a pitcher with baye Salte will become an Oyle, and is speciall good for Horses Legges strayned or brused, and may be applied for that purpose to anye other creature.

But an import from the New World, tobacco, was one of the wonder-drugs of its time. Here is Culpeper at his most lyrical:

> *Oyntment of Tobacco.* Joubertus.[15]
> Take of Tobacco leaves two pound; fresh Hogs grease diligently washed one pound; let the herb being bruised be infused a whol night in red Wine, in the morning let it boyl wth a gentle fire to the consumption of the Wine, strain it and ad to the Oyntment, of the juyce of Tobacco clarified half a pound; Rozin four ounces; boyl it to the consumption of the juyce, adding towards the end, round Birthwort roots in pouder two ounces, new Wax so much as is sufficient to make it into an Oyntment.
> A [Culpeper's added comment] It would ask a whol Summers day to write the particular vertues of this Oyntment, and my poor *Genius* is too weak to give it the hundreth [sic] part of its due praise, It cures Tumors, Aposthumes, Wounds, Ulcers, Gun-shot, Botches, Scabs, Itch, stinging with Nettles, Bees, Wasps, Hornets, venemous Beasts, Wounds made with poysoned Arrows &c. Tush! this is nothing – *paulo majora canamus.* It helps Scaldings though made with Oyl, Burnings though with Lightening, and that without any Scar: It helps nasty, rotten, stinking, putrefied Ulcers, though in the legs, whither the humors are most subject to resort; in Fistulaes though the bone be afflicted it shall scale it without any Instrument and bring up the flesh from the very bottom: Would you be fair? your face being anointed with this, soon will the Redness, Pimples, Sunburning vanish, a Wound dressed with this will never putrifie,

a Wound made with so small a weapon that no tent will follow [a roll of cloth used to keep wounds open], anoint but with this and you need fear no danger, If your head ach, anoint your temples with this and you shall have ease; The stomach being anointed with it, no infirmity dares harbor there, no not Asthmaes, nor consumptions of the lungues; The belly being anointed with it, helps the Chollick and Illiack passion, the Worms, and what not? it helps the Hemorrhoids or Piles, and is the best Oyntment that is, for gouts of all sorts: finally there may be as universal a medicine made for all diseases, of Tobacco as of any thing in the world, the *Philosophers Stone* excepted. O *Joubertus!* thou shalt never want praise for inventing this medicine, by those that use it, so long as the Sun and Moon endureth.

To say that tobacco was second only to the Philosopher's Stone was an enormous claim. The Stone was thought to be the culmination of years of patient work and unravelling of secrets. A pinch of the powder would transmute base metals such as lead into gold or silver, and an Elixir of Life could be prepared from it, which would cure all disease and give, if not actual immortality, many years above the normal span. If tobacco was almost, but not quite as good, it had the greater advantage of being more readily available. (It is ironic that Culpeper who died young of consumption, probably aggravated his illness by excessive tobacco smoking.)[16]

Joubertus was possibly a doctor or apothecary, but although the sun and moon are still in place, sadly he has slipped out of the firmament of fame.

'H. S.' one of the contributors to the later, Barrett manuscript, must have read this receipt, and been impressed enough to transcribe it into the notebook almost word for word, though she doesn't mention poor Joubertus, but shifts the credit to the donor of the ointment – 'you shall never want [lack] the prayers of those you give it to.'[17]

Internal injuries were difficult to treat because exploratory surgery was impossible. Probably the best that could be done was to give a medicine such as the Kidders', as full of healing herbs as could be gathered. It was not a first-aid measure though, because it took time to prepare. It must have been one you made and kept in case of need:

A Certain Receipte approved by Lady Newton

To make a drinke for [one] that is inwardly wounded cal'd a vulnerable pation [18]

Take scabious agrimone betonye wood Angelica senacle white bottle [?] planten ribwort dandelion wormwood sothernwood mugwort cumfrey buglosse speremint sinkefoyle strawberry leaues, vilott leaues red bramble leaues oake leaues hawthorne leaues or the younger topps thereof, woodbine leaues alens [sic] and Daysie leaues the roots and all; of each of these one handfull: boyle them in a gallon of spring water till ha[lf] the watter be boyled away then putt to [it] one quart of white wine then boyle it till one quart of the liquer be boyled away againe then straine the liquer from the herbes and put to it one pint of honye and boil itt till it be b[ut] a pottle then putt itt into some clean vessell and lett stand all night then power it from the dreggs and putt up into a cleane bottle then take of the drinke bloud warme 5 spoonfull in the morning and 4 in the afternoon about 4 of the Clocke.

With the blessing of Lady Newton perhaps the vulnerable patient recovered. It would all depend, of course, on the nature of the inward wound.

BLEEDING

Accidents with cutting tools, or sword-fights, could cause potentially fatal blood loss. William Harvey's discovery of the circulation of the blood was not available to the writers of early household books, but practical experience must have shown that compression was one way to stanch the flow. Cautery had been a cruel option too, until Ambroise Paré showed that gentler methods had better outcomes, but heat is still sometimes recommended for serious wounds.

Here are four suggestions by Thomas Dawson in about 1597:

For to Staunch Blood [19]

Take bole armoniake [a fine clay bought from the apothecary] and turpentine [resin], and make a plaster, and lay it to. Take the moss of the hazel tree and cast it into the wound, and it will staunch forthwith. The longer it is gathered the better it is. Also take a good piece of Martinmas beef out of the roast, and heat it on coals, and as hot as you may suffer it, lay it thereto. Also take a piece of lean salt beef, and let the beef be of that greatness that it may fill the wound, and lay it in the fire in the hot ashes till it be hot through, and all hot stuff it in the wound and bind it fast. And it shall staunch anon [soon] the bleeding when a master vein is cut, and if the wound be large.

Long-gathered or dried moss would have soaked up some of the blood from a smaller wound, and helped clotting. A different kind of very absorbent moss, sphagnum moss, was used as a dressing as recently as the First World War.[20] Perhaps growing on a hazel tree endowed it with special properties too. 'But each moss doth partake of the nature of the tree from whence it is taken' said Culpeper.[21] Mrs Corlyon has almost the same suggestion : 'Take of the greene mosse that groweth vppon an Hasell and lay it thicke vppon the wounde ...'[22]

Dawson's beef might have worked as well, though the idea of a hot dinner pushed into a gaping cut is not attractive nowadays. Perhaps better than bleeding to death though.

Other more puzzling receipts involve earthworms, frequently squashed and applied to heal wounds. They were used therapeutically for hundreds of years. Dioscorides said that when beaten small and applied to an injury they joined sinews that had been cut. The *Leechbook of Bald* has precisely the same advice.[23] The thirteenth-century MS BL Sloane 145 has the same for a man with cut nerves.[24]

Mrs Corlyon then was hardly being original in this receipt:

A Medecine to stanche bleedinge to knytt the Synnowes and to heale any greene wounde hauing no Boone perished [25]
Tak[e] the longe wormes of the earthe commonly called knott wormes stampe them and spreade them very thicke vppon a clothe and so lay them to the wounde Note that so longe as it cleauethe you must not take it of[f] but if it falleth of[f] then must you applye more of them to the wounde. This taken in tyme will heale it in 8. or 9 dayes.

The persistence of this belief may involve sympathetic magic. Earthworms can grow new segments at the tail end if they are damaged, so perhaps their flesh might have been thought to cause renewal in others.

Mrs Corlyon also has an odd cure for a severe nosebleed:

> An other Medecine for Bleedinge at the Nose that will assuredlye helpe, if all other do fayle [26]
> Make a Plaister of Pitche vppon Leather and laye it betwixte your shoulders colde, and lett your Plaister be cutt to couer the one halfe of your Shoulder blades and so goe smale vpwardes to the nape of your necke and lay an other of the same to the Reynes of your Backe [the kidney area] and these togeather vndoubtedlye will staye [stop] your Bleedinge

Undoubtedly? Maybe the shock of cold pitch might do something … (There is a folklore cure in recent memory of dropping a cold key down the back.) She repeats the treatment in a searcloth for pain in the spleen, or a stitch or wind. 'It is good also to stanche Bleedinge.'[27] This time the pitch is melted and spread on leather before application to the same areas.

BURNS AND SCALDS

Again, there was a diversity of cures. Lucastella's Balsam was an elaborate panacea (see p. 53) but easier ones were possibly just as effective. Mrs Corlyon, who was hot on burn treatments, so to speak, has several salves, ointments and other dressings. Ground ivy was good for burns in this receipt (it was also known as alehoof, and used for clearing beer):

> A Salue good to cure any Burninge or Scalding [28]
> Take a good quantitye of grounde Iuye [Ivy], stampe it well, then let it boile in a sufficient quantitye of Deares sewett ouer a softe fyer vntill it looketh blacke, then straine it and keepe it in a Caake as longe as you please.

> When you will vse it melte a little in a sawser and with a feather
> annoynte the place.

A feather was often suggested to apply ointments to a hurt. It would
get it onto the injured part without further damage.

A cerecloth would have been a practical treatment for larger areas
of burnt skin. It is basically a waxed or greased cloth – the word
comes from the Latin, *cera*, wax. The same kind of cloths were used
as winding-sheets for the dead, but have no particularly sinister
associations in the medical receipts. As they were waterproof they
would have excluded air too, which is an important consideration
in reducing the pain of burns:

> A very good Seareclothe for all manner of heate for any Burninge,
> or Scaldinge, or to asswage the Heate about any Soore[29]
> Take of Deares sewett, of Maye Butter, Capons grease Oyle of Roses
> Honnye, Waxe Allome and redd Rose water of all these a prettye
> quantitye accordinge to discretion. Add to all these a quantitye of
> the iuyce of Houselicke, sett them on the fyer and lett them boile
> togeather a quarter of an hower or better Then straine it through a
> cleane clothe and after dipp your clothes into it and smothe them well
> with your handes against the fyer and when it is colde, folde it vpp
> and keepe it for your vse. One Searecloth will serue 4. dayes if you
> wipe it cleane it cleane [sic] euery dressinge and lay on the other syde.

Oil of roses and rose water are soothing, honey is antiseptic (our
term) and houseleek had been famous since ancient times as a cure
for burns, good for many skin complaints, too. (It could even be
said to be a preventative of burns, in that it protects the house on
which it grows from lightning.[30]) Easy to grow, quick to multiply,
it is an extremely useful fleshy little plant, tough and resistant to
drought. No roof should be without one.

Mrs Corlyon evidently valued her cerecloth more than we might
consider hygienic, as you could simply wipe it down and turn it
over to re-apply.

Firearms were another cause of injury both early and late in the
seventeenth century. First is Mrs Corlyon again:

A Salue for any wounde caused by Gunshott[31]

First if by any meanes you can gett out the shott, but whether you can
or no dresse it in this manner. Take a pinte of Venice Turpentine as
much of the Oyle of Lynseede, a quarter of an ownze of Verdegrease
beaten into fyne powder. Lett these boile togeather one wame [just
brought to boil] then straine them and putt it vpp close and vse it
thus Warme it and dipp lynt in it and so applye it to the wounde,
and besides poure some of it warmed into the wounde But for any
manner of wounde in the Heade: Take a quantitye of Aquavite and
putt into it Sugar and therewith thoroughlye washe the wounde
and stoppe it up with lynt dipped therein. And dresse it thus once
in 24. howers.

Not much had changed seventy years later regarding the *semper-
vivum tectorum*, or houseleek, but dung makes an appearance in
Hannah Woolley's receipt of 1675. Dung had been used in some
Anglo-Saxon receipts, and the idea was evidently persistent, as it is
applied to a 'new' type of injury:

A very good receipt for one hurt with Gun-powder.[32]

Take twelve heads of Housleek, one handful of Groundsel, one pint
of Goose-dung, as much Chicken-dung of the newest that can be
gotten; stamp the Herbs very small, then put the dung into a Mortar,
temper them together with a pottle of Bores-grease, stir them together half an hour, then strain it through a Canvas-bag and so
preserve it for your use; it will keep two years, and be not the worse.

Boar's grease was lard, very often used as a basis for ointments.
Whether it would really have lasted for two years without going
off is doubtful.

BITES FROM VENOMOUS AND OTHER BEASTS

Culpeper's (and Barrett's) ointment made from tobacco, given
above, would take care of most emergencies of this kind, but if
you had none there were alternatives.

'Venemous beasts' are frequently mentioned, and may include hornets, wasps and bees. For wasp stings *The Queen's Closet* suggests 'a little Plaister of Treacle'[33] that is Venice or London Treacle, presumably.

In this country the adder is the only native venomous creature. Mrs Corlyon had an interesting group of receipts to deal with adder bite.[34] It has been suggested that she was a Cornishwoman.[35] As adders are common in the West Country she may have had first-hand knowledge of them. Adder bites cause pain and swelling, and even death, but this is rare. Children may be affected more severely than adults:

> A Medecine for the stynginge of an Edder.
> Take a Cocke and cleaue [cleave] hym in the middest so soone as he is killed the feathers beyinge vppon hym and laye hym to the place guttes and all before he be colde, and so lett hym lye 7. howers or 8. and then lay an other in the same sorte and it will helpe And withall geue the Patient Tryackle to drincke to keepe the poyson from the Harte.

Using newly killed poultry as a heat source was common to several treatments. On a farm it might be easier to get hold of a bird for immediate application than to mess about in the kitchen heating ingredients for a poultice. There also seems to have been a belief that poison could be drawn out of the body by a bird, as in the Queen's plague medicine on p. 98. Tryackle, that is theriac or treacle, was a universal antidote to poison, described more fully on p. 55. If you had no cockerels handy you could use herbs instead:

> An other Medecine for one that is stonge with an Edder.
> Take Mustarde Seede and bruse it in a woodden dishe with Dragon Water then openinge the wounde with a fyne Needle (first bynding the Patient about the place where he is hurte for swellinge eny further) Bathe the Wounde and all about as farr as it is swelled with the Dragon water and then lay the Medecine on the wounde byndinge it on with a fayre clothe: And when you dress it againe annoynte it with Oyle of Roses: Geue the Patient Tryackle and Dragon water to drincke when you dress it firste.

Opening the punctured skin with a needle and bandaging above and below the wound were no doubt attempts to expel the venom and stop it spreading. Treacle was given, as in the first remedy. The dragon water was most likely made from gum tragacath, also known as gum dragon, but could possibly be made from Culpeper's Dragon, *Dracontium* (too well known to need a description, unfortunately), but 'it is excellent good against pestilence and poison. Pliny and Dioscorides affirm, that no serpent will meddle with him that carries the herb about him.' If so, it was a pity that the victim couldn't find it before the encounter, rather than afterwards:

> An other Medecine for the stynginge of an Edder or Snake or any other venemous thinge
> Take a good quantitye of St John's woorte and stampe it well, putt thereto a good prettye quantitye of the best wine Vinegar you can gett and so applye it to the place that is so stonge and it will presently drawe out the venome and cure it. And for any Beaste that is stonge about the Vdder or any other parte take rotten Egges (w[hi]ch it wilbe good to keepe alwayes in a readynesse in some pott. Beate the Egges well togeather, and rubb and chafe the place well for a good space togeather and it will presentlye cure any such stinginge or venominge eyther in Man or Beaste.

Culpeper approves of St John's wort as a wound herb (as in Mrs Corlyon's ointment above), and 'good for those that are bitten or stung by any venomous creature.' (It is now being used as an anti-depressant.) Mrs Corlyon, evidently a countrywoman, was concerned about farm beasts too, and mention of the [cow's] udder ties in with an old idea that adders sucked milk from cows.[36] In adder-infested areas keeping rotten eggs in readiness is reminiscent of the anti-venin stores of modern hospitals. One can only hope they were kept downwind in an outhouse though.

More conventionally, *The Queen's Closet* resorts to hazel nuts, with rue, garlic and treacle the well-known antidotes to poison of any kind. Evidently, the snake venom, and 'venom' from the mad dog were thought to be similar. Another receipt on the same page gives mashed garlic as a remedy against snakebite in general. The veterinary concern appears here as well:

> For the biting of a madde Dogge or stinging of an Adder.[37]
> Take a handful or more of hazle Nuts, a quarter as much of Rue, with a clove of Garlick, stamp all these together, then take the juyce, and put a little Treacle to it, and if it be a man that is stung or bitten, give it him to drink in Beer or Wine, or Ale; but if a Dog, give it in Milk; then take that from whence the juyce came, and bind it to the place which was bit or stung.

Some variation was made by Mrs Miller in 1660. Her cure for the bite of a mad dog still included rue, garlick, and Venice treacle, but now added 'scrap'd Tin or the best pewter.'[38] Made into a decoction with ale or beer, the dose was eight to nine spoonfuls on an empty stomach for three days. It could also be given in smaller doses to dog, hog or sheep – even to a baby. 'The gentleman that recommended this receipt never knew it fail man or Beast, if taken within nine days after the Bite.' Maybe the dog was mad from some other cause than rabies?

However, rabies – hydrophobia – does seem to be implicated in another receipt in the same collection.[39] 'A certain cure' involves bleeding the patient in the old Galenic way, then taking a powder of 'ash-coloured ground Liverwort [a lichen] and black pepper', with milk. Fear of water evidently had to be overcome, so the receipt continues:

> ... the Patient must go into the cold Bath or a cold spring or River ev'ry morning fasting for a month: He must be dip't all over, but not stay in (with his Head above water) longer than half a minute if the water be very cold. After this he must go in three times a week for a fortnight longer.

An animal did not need to be mad to have a troublesome bite. Mrs Corlyon had a salve for almost everything, including the

'Bytinge of a Dogge, a Hogge a Horse or a Man.'[40] (She does not elaborate on the circumstances of a human bite.) The cure anyway was chopped ragwort, boiled to a green salve with fresh butter.

Of all the manuscript collections I have looked at, Mrs Corlyon is the clear leader in receipts to cope with accidents of all kinds. She gives the impression of being coolly in command – according to the standards of her times, of course. One can only admire her and any other women called on to set bones, stop serious bleeding, reduce the shock and hurt of burns, deal with gunshot wounds, and cope with the attacks of angry beasts and adders. Quick intervention would have saved many lives, even if not all.

5

Fevers and Frets

FEVERS IN GENERAL AND AGUE IN PARTICULAR

Galen had thought that fevers resulted from an excess of any one of the four humours. They might then cause putrefaction and too much heat. Blood-letting was the cure.[1] Theory had moved on from this in the seventeenth century, but not much. Fever and ague tended to be lumped together, but many diseases now had specific names. Plague for instance, and spotted fever, were perceived as separate conditions. Dr Thomas Willis, also a pioneer on the structure and functions of the brain, wrote an influential book on fevers in the mid-fifties. Thomas Sydenham stressed observation and experience in treating diseases such as smallpox. But even after this, household manuscripts took little notice of controversial theories. A fever was a fever. The home practitioner really only wanted to know what to do for it, not what caused it.

Mrs Corlyon has only a few treatments for fever as such, but her nursing was careful. A broth for 'an hott Feuer'[2] is a pleasant jelly made from veal and mutton bones with herbs and dried fruit. She has a herbal mixture to induce sweating to be taken before an attack of ague was expected.[3] Another remedy for ague involved an ointment with chopped herbs bound to the wrists.[4] More such wrist treatments are described below.

Other manuscripts also suggest palliative care. This drink would do no harm at least:

A Julipp for a Burninge Feauer[5]
Take a pinte of Barley water two sponfull of sirrop of Lemons and eight spoonfull of white wine good.

AGUE

Markham summed up the fever/ague problem.[6] He remarks 'Of feuers in generall' that the common ones are quotidian, tertian and quartan agues. Another sort was an accidental fever 'which commeth by meanes of some dangerous wound receiued'. Additionally 'There be sundry other feuers which, comming from consumptions, and other long continued sicknesses, doe altogether surpasse our Hus-wiues capacity.' However he went on to tell her what to do for the hectic fever (a mixture of oil of violets and ground white poppy seed rubbed into the back), pestilent fever and plague.

The bracketing together of ague and fever occurs too in the Bills of Mortality, where even in the plague year of 1665 there were 5,257 deaths in London from these causes. (Plague of course accounted for far more.)

The different sorts of ague are now thought to have been forms of malaria. (This name comes from the Italian, *mal aria*, bad air, with an ancient connection to swampy places.) The female *Anopheles* mosquito can carry a small parasite, any one of four types of *Plasmodium* protozoa, which get transferred to the human victim of her bloodsucking bite. An infected person in turn passes the parasite back to another mosquito. Once inside the human body, the parasites multiply and break out of the blood cells in regular peaks, causing attacks of shivering and sweating. If it lasts more than a day it is called *quotidian*, according to Markham, coming every other day, *tertian*, and every third day *quartan* fever. (Not what you would expect. A day seems to have got lost somewhere.)

Sometimes there may be infection from several different kinds of parasites, when the distinction breaks down. Because it is basically a disease of the liver and blood, the patient may become anaemic and develop jaundice, stomach complaints, and other ills. In the household books jaudice is treated as a separate disease, and of course may be caused by other liver conditions, but many cases probably had their origin in ague.

Treatments in the first half of the century were probably ineffectual. Markham's include eating an egg yolk mixed with aqua vitae, and then sweating the fever out, or a decoction of dandelion, and

work until you sweat. The dandelion is diuretic too. He recognised
that quartan fever or third day ague was dangerous, 'because many
times consumptions, blacke iaundies and such like mortall sicknesses
follow it.' The treatment was with mithridate and lemon – not taken
internally, as might be reasonable, but 'so as the lemman be couered
with the mithridate; then bind it to the pulse of the sickemans wrist
of his arme about an houre before his fit doth beginne.' He was then
allowed to take hot posset ale and mithridate after sweating. Sweating
was seen as a way of getting rid of whatever was causing disease.

This is not the only wrist cure. Markham has a herbal paste to
apply 'For any Feuer'.[7] The Barrett manuscript contains a herbal
cure 'For a tertian ague, p[re]scribed to my wife in the spring, after
3. or 4. fits. By her father'.[8] The writer, Francis Head, adds a sceptical
note: 'If she have anie faith in wrest plaisters, she may make them
of Bole Armenic [a medicinal clay], white frankincense powdered
and venice turpentine.'

Lemons turn up on several other occasions too. This, which we
should call lemonade, is like the julip for fever above:

Doctor Shirrod for an ague for an ancient body[9]
Take 3 lemones and slice them rines an meate together then put them
in a pottle of spring water and boyle it to a quart then take it from the
fire an put it in a stone pott and put to it a quarter of a pound of loafe
suger an let the pacient drink of this at all times and no other drinke

At some time between 1630 and 1640 a new herbal medicine was
brought from the New World. It was called cinchona or Peruvian
bark, also known as Jesuits' Bark because they recognised its value.
It was a source of quinine, a really effective remedy against malaria,
though there was prejudice against it – too Catholic for Protestants,
too 'hot' for Galenists. However, it does find its way into the later
household books, one of the few signs that things were changing.
Here is Mrs Miller in 1660:

To Infuse the Bark for an ague[10]
Take a pint of water and boil it and put into it an ounce of Bark
when its almost cold. Then mix it with a pint of Claret, and drink a

quarter of a pint at a time once in four hours when the Hot fit and cold fit is quite off.

JAUNDICE

There could be many reasons for jaundice, including repeated attacks of ague. The yellow tinge to skin and eyes is just a symptom of liver problems. In the household manuscripts two kinds predominate, 'black' and/or 'yellow'. Mrs Corlyon devoted a whole chapter of eleven receipts to the condition,[11] plus a few others such as a 'Snayle water'.[12]

Almosts all the receipts in her main chapter include saffron, turmeric or 'yeollowe rootes of Dockes', most probably an indication of the Doctrine of Signatures, where herbs had some point in common with the organ or disease being treated, in this case the colour. (This is true of many manuscripts.) Others have the archaic ingredients of animal dung or earthworms, and the magical ones of ivory, stag's or unicorn horns. (More about these in Chapter 12.)

This receipt is one of the most benign:

An other Medecine for those that ar enteringe into the yeollowe Iaundyes[13]
Take a good rostinge Aple, cutt of the topp of it and take out the coore, then fyll it vpp with the powder of Turmericke or of Stagges horne, and a litle Saffron, then sett on the toppe and roste it very softe, and when it is rosted wringe it out vppon a Sawser and scrape Sugar thereon, and eate so much euery morninge for 8. or 9. dayes and it will helpe.

The Barrett manuscript, in contrast, goes to bizarre lengths:

For a black Jaundise[14]
Slit a tench in the middle, & tye the same (guts and all) crosse the stomach, for the space of 24. hours. The next day applie another. This will be noysom & troublesom, but hath proued [proved] effectual to diuerse [several people].

After a couple of days of this, the jaundice may have seemed less of a problem by comparison.

Frets – Eyes

Eye problems could afflict anyone. Pepys was so troubled that he was forced to abandon his diary. John Milton went blind. To most people the threat of loss of sight must have been terrifying. No wonder then that there are very many receipts devoted to sight. Conditions identified in the manuscript and printed books include styes, sore eyes, bleared eyes, redness, pain, pearl, pin and web, rheum and blood in the eye, dimness of sight, cataract, flesh in the corner of the eye, bruise and burns from fire or gunpowder. There are medicines to comfort the sight, to clear it, preserve or restore it, and to defend from humours. However, I have found no reference to spectacles, though the London Guild of Spectacle Makers was established in 1629.

Styes were perhaps the least serious frets, but could be painful. An early receipt from Grace Acton's little manuscript of 1621 uses slightly exotic ingredients:

> For a Sty on the eye.[15]
> Take hedghogge lard and verdigris and mix wythe asses milk in a silver pot apply to the eye with a hares tail.

The hare's tail was soft, a method of applying ointment gently. A feather could be used in the same way.

As mentioned before, Mrs Corlyon's book is well organised. The 'Eyes' chapter has twenty-six receipts. It is the first in the book, as she was following a medieval top-to-toe order of bodily parts, more or less.

Sometimes the eye could be generally sore, no reason given, so a herbal cure could be tried. It was good for man or beast:

> A Medecine for a sore Eye[16]
> Take Pearle woorte, stampe and straine and myngle the iuyce therof with woemans milke and white Sugar candye powdered, and so

droppe it into the Eye Take also Ribbwoorte, and if it be needfull
to washe it, lett it be well dryed from the water then stampe and
straine it, and dropp a good droppe thereof 2. or 3. tymes a daye into
the eye. This of Ribbwoorte is also good for any Beastes or Cattell
that have Soore eyes.

Ribwort was a country name for plantain, easy to find, and free.

Various different simples were recommended. The Parker manuscript has another suggestion 'for sore eyes take celindine and distill
and drope into the eyes 3. or four times a day.'[17] The Barrett manuscript uses plain expressed juice in 'A medison for Sore Eyes. Take
the juce of fenill & drop it in the eyes, evenings & mornings & it will
heal them. H. S.' (H. S. was one of the possibly female contributors
to this manuscript.) It is an easy and practical receipt. Gerarde gives
a couplet under his entry 'Of Fennel':[18]

> Of Fennell, Roses, Vervain, Rue and Celandine,
> Is made a water good to cleere the sight of eine.

In his account of ground ivy,[19] he says:

> Ground-Ivy, Celandine, and Daisies, of each a like quantitie,
> stamped and strained, and a little sugar and rose water put thereto,
> and dropped with a feather into the eies, taketh away all maner of
> inflammation, spots, webs, itch, smarting, or any griefe whatsoever
> in the eyes, yea although the sight were nigh hand gone: it is proved
> to be the best medicine in the world.

The same herbs mixed with ale and honey, and strained, could also
be used to 'take away the pinne and web, or any griefe out of the
eyes of horse or cow, or any other beast.'

Pin and web was a common complaint, appearing in all the printed
and manuscript collections. It seems to have been a spreading film
or opaque area starting from a single point in the eye. The remedies
are varied however, without much consensus on treatment. Mrs
Corlyon's remedies include mashed slugs[20] as well as this one, which
is rather more appealing, though possible no more effective:

An other Medecine for to take away the Pynn and webb in the eye, or a Tey in the eye, w[hi]ch growethe from the corner of the eye to the blacke, and is like a litle Gutt.[21]

Take of fyne white Sugar as much as a Wallnutt, and a peece of Sanguis Draconis [dragon's blood, a gum] as bigg as a Beane, and beate them togeather very fyne; Searze [sift] it throughe a peece of Lawne, and putt a litle of this powder into your eye euening, morning, and at midd tyme of the daye, and slumber a litle after, and by Gods helpe it will cure.

The Queen's Closet agrees that dragon's blood can help aching or red eyes,[22] but offers a laconic and painful receipt for the more serious condition:

For a Pin or Web in the Eye far gone.[23]
Take the Marrow of a Goose wing, and mingle the powder of Ginger therewith, dress the Eye therewith two or three times a day.

Once blind, the case is desperate. Remedies get more far-fetched and claims of cures more strident. The Parker manuscript has 'a very pretious water for the eyes' [24] which uses a lot of herbs: smallage, fennel, rue, agrimony, betony, sabious, sage, and pimpernell, distilled with 'a little uring of a childe and 5 graines of frankensence'. This was dripped into the eyes every night, 'and they shall have sight God willing.' Perhaps the child's urine was thought to be both pure and regenerative.

Markham includes eyebright – euphrasia – fennel and celandine for another precious medicine:

A precious water for the eyes.[25]
Take of *Red rose leaues*, of *Smallage* of maidenhair, *Eusaace* [sic, eufrace or euphrasia], *endiue, succory, red fennell, hill-wort*, and *cellandine*, of each halfe a quarter of a pound, wash them cleene and lay them in steepe in white wine a whole day, then still them in an ordinary still, & the first water will be like gold, the second like siluer, and the third like balme: any of theese is most pretious for sore eyes, and hath recouered sight lost for the space of Ten yeares, having been vsed but foure dayes.

Were such claims believed, or merely hoped for? One receipt from Mrs Miller's collection suggests that someone was adding a little irony to her ink. It is 'A Receipt to Clear the eyes found out by Dr Purolon [?] Bishop of Hull who could See better at the Age of 125 than at 50 by the use of this Medicine'[26] It is based on the 'Oyle of a white of an Egg' – but egg whites contain no oil whatever. According to the receipt, egg whites well beaten and left for six hours will separate into an oil and residual froth.

Frets – Ears

Compared with eye disease, the ears get much less attention in the household books. Mrs Corlyon gives only six receipts in her chapter on Ears; three of those are for tinnitis, and all deliver steam into the ear.[27] The first is a poultice of hot barley bread, sprinkled with nutmeg and held to the ear, another uses ground ivy and pennyroyal boiled in sack. 'Lett the steeme thereof goo into your eares by a tunnell that will close couer the pott.' The third is for a big onion, stuffed with mithridate, salad oil and aquavitae, wrapped in paper and roast. When soft it is mashed, laid on a cloth, and held to the ear as hot as the patient can bear it.

Earwax can build up and cause deafness, and Mrs Corlyon treats this too with steam and oil.[28]

According to Gerarde, ground ivy was also good for 'the humming noyse and ringing sound of the eares, being put into them, and for them that are hard of hearing.'[29]

The Parker manuscript gets in first (1651) with a receipt 'for on[e] that is thicke of hearing',[30] before W.M. of *The Queen's Closet* (1655).[31] Juice of garden daisy roots is dropped into the ear – but, mysteriously, on the *better* side. If this is a mistake, it is repeated. The dosage was three or four drops, either for 2–3 or 3–4 days.

Mrs Corlyon, never at a loss, and evidently living close to an orchard, had the answer to another hazard:

A Medecine to drawe an Earewigge out of the Eare[32]

Take a sweete Aple and rost it in the fyer vntill it bee halfe rosted, then take of the softest of it, and spreade it very thick vppon a lynnen clothe, and lay it to your eare as hott as you can suffer it, and lye vppon the same syde, and when you do feele it stirr, you must lye very still vntill it be come to the Aple, and then you must very sodainly pluck it away least the Earewigge retorne into youre heade againe. And if you thinke there be any more laye a newe one to your eare.

Later, Gervase Markham had a different remedy for unwelcome visitors:

For any venom in the eare.[33]
Take the iuice of *Louage* and drop it into the eare, and it will cure any venome, and kill any worme, earewigge, or other vermine.

FRETS – TEETH

Dental hygiene was not well developed, though some tooth-cleaning was done, by methods given on p. 178. The black smiles of Elizabethan ladies who ate too much sugar are well known. Even the Queen had painful teeth. The tooth-drawer at a fair is the stereotype of the quack doctor or mountebank, putting on a show and selling his patent medicines at the same time. Nevertheless, pulling out a rotten tooth must have given relief, no matter who did it.

Mrs Corlyon, as usual, covers several aspects of care. Prevention was better than cure of course. However, scrubbing the teeth was not to be overdone:

A Medecine to skower the teethe, to make them cleane and stronge, and to preserue them from perishinge beyng vsed two or three tymes a weeke.[34]
Take of Currall [coral] and of Amber fynely beaten of eche a like quantity. Blend these with as much Honny as will serue to make it like a Conserue: Temper these well togeather then putt them in a glasse and keepe it for your vse and when you doo vse it take a litle of it vppon a course clothe and rubb your teeth therewith . As much as a Barlye corne will serue for all your teethe.

It was obvious that sometimes small holes appeared in the teeth nevertheless, so the reasonable conclusion was that little worms had caused them. Mrs Corlyon had one medicine to 'drawe downe the Rhewme, if it be a worme it will kill it.' A bad pain could be eased by the (poisonous and dangerous) narcotic of henbane:

An other Medecine for the Toothe ache[35]
Take an Henbane roote, scrape it and washe it cleane, then slyce it, and boyle it in a good quantity of wine Vineger and three spoonefulles of Rose water, boile these togeather in a Platter uppon a chafingdish of coales vntill the vinegar be consumed that it will scarce couer the rootes then take it of, and take one of the Slyces and holde it betwixt your teeth somewhat warme vppon the toothe that dothe ake, and take a litle of the lyquor in your mouthe warme and leane your heade vppon the Syde that your greefe is, and after that you haue holden it in your mouthe about halfe an hower, hauing chaunged it twice or thryce in that tyme putt it out and do this as you shall feele occasion and you shall fynde ease. Probatum est.

True, she tells the patient to 'putt it out', that is spit, don't swallow, but it would be difficult not to let some of it slip down by accident.

Milder measures could be tried too. The Barrett manuscript suggests sniffing the juice of small daisy roots 'into the contrarie nostrell', or making a paste of powdered ginger and egg white to apply to the face on the aching side.[36]

A counter-irritant might do the trick. Perhaps the idea in this one was to draw the pain downwards:

For the Toothache[37]
Spread Burgamy=Pitch on Leather. Strew the plaister with Nutmeg, and Lay it on warm to the Souls of your feet. Let it be on as long as it will stick Doctor Gardener

It is unlikely that such palliatives cured the toothache permanently however. There came a time when the tooth had to go, either by being pulled out with pincers or by other means. You could try Markham's method:

To draw teeth without yron[38]
Take some of the greene of the elder tree, or the apples of oake trees
and with either of these rub the teeth and gummess and it will loosen
them so as you may take them out.

Another way given by Hannah Woolley was to fill the cavity of
the tooth with spurge juice and wheat flour, changing it every two
hours until the tooth dropped out. Spurge is a strong caustic so
it might have done as she says. She may have got the idea from
Gerarde, who also states the juice may be put into hollow teeth,
'being put into them warily, so that you touch neither the gums,
nor any of the other teeth in the mouth with the said medicine.'[39]
Spurge was not a remedy he would recommend though, as there
were better alternatives.

The books hardly mention them, but false teeth were available,
made from ivory or bone, or by courtesy of battlefield casualties.

Frets of the Skin

The skin is the barrier between a rough unfriendly environment and
the inner smooth working of the body. In the developed world we
now generally have the privilege of a clean water supply, effective
soap, shampoo, toothpaste, and habits of using them. It is routine to
cover all but the most minor scratches if the skin is broken. We take
measures to remove fleas, lice, and bugs from our houses, clothes
and persons. 'Progress' can be an elusive thing, but personal hygiene
does qualify.

The seventeenth-century epidermis must have been a general
mess if the number of receipts for skin treatments indicates the
extent of disease. Cosmetic aspects of skin complaints will come in
a later chapter, but here are some of the more serious and painful
afflictions and their remedies.

Spots could turn to boils, felons or whitlows, boils to abscesses or
imposthumes. Serious abscesses could form fistulas – ulcers like tun-
nels eating into the flesh. Scabs, old scars and sores of all kinds needed
salves and ointments to heal and dry them. Morphew, ringworm

and itch, and the King's Evil were decided frets. (Syphilis caused sores too: see p. 100) Leprosy is mentioned, but was becoming rare.

Kitchen physic is sometimes difficult to distinguish from kitchen cookery. The housewife used what was to hand for common complaints, such as boils. This one would probably have been a perfectly good dressing (or breakfast):

> A Medecine for a pushe or a Byle[40]
> Take of grated crummes of white Breade a quantitye of Milke and some English Saffron, make thereof a Pultesse and apply it warme, it will rypen breake drawe and heale.

Markham's poultice is similar, with the addition of herbs:

> A pultus to drie a sore.[41]
> To drie vp any sore, take Smalledge [wild celery], Groundsell, wilde mallowes, and violet leaues: chop them small and boile them in milke with bruised oatmeale and sheeps suet, and so apply it to the sore.

Oil of egg yolks was a useful standby for the medicine shelf. Markham suggests it for burns[42] and so does *The Queen's Closet*.[43] Culpeper gives it in his *Dispensatory* with his comments on multiple uses. It was not to be taken internally, but applied where it would do most good:

> *Oyl of the Yolks of Egs.* Mesue[44]
> Take of the Yolks of Egs boyled hard, warm them well with a gentle fire in a glazed vessel, but have a care you burn them not, then press out the Oyl with a press, and if whilst they are warming, you sprinkle them with a little Wine, the Oyl will come out the better.

> It is profitable in fistulaes and malignant ulcers, it causeth the hair to grow, it cleers the skin and takes away deformities thereof, viz. Tatters, Ringworms, Morphew, Scabs. I suppose none is so simple to take it inwardly to cleer their skin, nor to anoint their feet to take away the deformity of their face.

Some people *were* inclined to take medicine inwardly to clear the skin, and a strange (but not unique) mix it might be:

a medesin for an impostume in the body[45]
take stone hors dunge that coms from the hors which is keept at hous and eateth no grase but provender, take a handfull of it as fresh as you can get it if it be hott from the hors soe much the beter and strayne it with white wine and drinke it every morning

Cures for the itch and ringworm were more rational and possibly effective. The itch was probably scabies, infestation by a small parasitic mite which burrows into the skin. It causes severe itching, leading to scratching, causing sores and scabs.

Mrs Corlyon has help for 'an Itche that hath been of longe continuance'[46] which involves first drinking stale beer with added madder (as in the cure for syphilis on p. 101), but which goes on:

And withall lett the partye euery morning sytt naked before a good fyer, and lett hym be well rubbed all over his Bodye and so the heate of the fyer and the rubbinge will make the Itche to come out Then take a smoothe sticke flatt, and annoynte the Bodye very thyn over with Tarre beynge moulten with freshe grease or Sheepes tallow beynge tryed, and lett hym not putt on his clothes till he be drye. This doe by the space of 12. dayes and it will helpe.

The tar could have killed the parasite, though it would have been unpleasant to go around for twelve days with skin sticky and smelling like old rope. Quicksilver could also be applied.[47] Brimstone was an alternative ingredient, as in Hannah Woolley's receipt:

Against the Itch.[48]
Take sweet Butter, unwrought Wax, Vinegar, Brimstone, a little Rose-water & red Cloves whole, boil them together till they be like Salve, then anoint the fleshe three sundry nights by the fire therewith, and no more, and you need not question a cure.

Ringworm is caused by a fungus, leading to itchy scaly patches. Like scabies, it is contagious. Markham cures it by applying bruised celandine, picked early in the morning. The flowers do not open before nine o'clock,[49] so there may be a hint of magic here – maybe the closed flowers caused the ringworm to contract? Celandine is used frequently in other remedies for the skin anyway.

Warts have been a staple of folklore, because there are so many country cures for them. They are caused, apparently, by a virus, but can appear and disappear in a magical manner, though some may be very persistent. Oliver Cromwell possessed the most famous set in history, having his portrait painted 'warts and all', presumably to show that he didn't mind being seen with human imperfections. We don't know if he tried to get rid of them or not, but in his travels round the country he could have taken his choice of treatments. Susan Drury's thesis[50] covers a multitude of plants and ailments, not just wart cures, but it does include a fair number of these. For example, apple slices (North Country), or stolen bacon (Suffolk) could be rubbed on, and then allowed to decay. Also in Suffolk, Cromwell could have carved his initials into an ash tree, and as the bark healed so would his blemishes. In the West Country applying buttercup or crowsfoot sap might have done it. Back in the North, in Yorkshire, he could have thrown bad peas, each representing a single wart, over his left shoulder, and ridden off without looking back. Anywhere he could have found honeysuckle or onions to make poultices, or common poppy, rue, spurge or marigolds for their sap. However, one cure, to bind slices of potato to the affected part, might not have made him look like a role-model for his New Army. Better keep the warts, after all.

THE KING'S EVIL

Here we step across a boundary between natural and supernatural cures. The disease was natural enough, now known as scrofula. It is a tubercular infection of bones and lymphatic glands, particularly those of the neck, resulting in painful sores like boils, and potentially fatal. Yet for some reason it had been singled out for a type of faith-healing, a laying-on of hands by the reigning monarch. Hence the name. In England the practice had begun with Edward the Confessor. It was enthusiastically carried out by King Charles I, who saw in it a further confirmation of his Divine Right to rule. Charles II also 'touched'. On 23 June 1660, Pepys went to see the ceremony. But the king 'did not come at all, it rayned so; and the poor people were forced to stand all the morning in the rain in the garden. Afterwards, he touched them in the Banquetting-house.'[51] As well as the royal touch, the sufferers were given a coin, to be worn as an amulet.

Perhaps, if the king turned up, the royal charm worked in some cases. It must have been flattering to have the sovereign himself condescending to stroke your painful neck. The mind can sometimes perform apparent miracles of healing. Maybe some people had natural remissions too. This was long before statistical evaluation of treatments, but royal touching certainly survived as a custom until the accession of George I.

However, some household books recognised that the king's hand might not always cure. The Barrett manuscript has a water 'to cure A Fistula, The Kings Evil, when touching it would not doe it.'[52] The Evil may be treated simply as a swelling, and the medicines for it used for other things too. Here is one of Mrs Corlyon's poultices:

A good Medecine for the Kinges Evell so that it be taken at the beginninge. And it is good for any other swelling in the throote or in any other part of the bodye[53]

Take a pretty quantitye of the slyces of course breade eyther of wheate or Rye that is stronge of the leauen, and an handfull of dried redd Rose leaves. Boile these in a quart of Beere and when it groweth somewhat thicke putt thereto 4. or 5. spoonefulles of Englishe honnye, and with a clothe applye it warme to the place greeued, after 12 howers shifte it and apply freshe and it will helpe.

A wide-spectrum ointment, added in a different hand, was based on the standby Venice turpentine (see p. 53). It could be 'giuen both inwardly and outwardly for the kinges evil for the plurisy, bur[n] ings, scaldings green wounds, & sore eyes.'[54]

Markham has a specific remedy, however.[55] Red dock is boiled in wine until tender, the liquid strained, and a 'good draught thereof' taken. Continued use is recommended. Culpeper says that red dock, also known as bloodwort, 'is exceeding strengthening to the liver, and procures good blood ...' so we seem to be back to humoral theory, with the king's evil seen as a defect of the blood. Maybe the red colour of the dock made it special too.

Rest and nursing care with cooling drinks or nourishing broths would have gone a long way to helping the body heal itself in fevers – with luck, and if God willed it. The frets were sources of discomfort and malfunction. Poor sight, loss of hearing, bad teeth and painful skin conditions were not immediately fatal, but were things to be endured, with as much help from herbs, poultices and ointments as the compassionate housewife could produce from her garden, storeroom or shopping trip to the apothecary in town. You might even get the king himself to intervene while you were at it.

6

Desperate Diseases: Plague, Poxes and Consumption

PLAGUE

The plague returned at intervals to kill large numbers of people after its first appearance in England as the Black Death. The main epidemics of the seventeenth century were those of 1603, 1625, an outbreak during the Civil War (as if there were not enough horrors already), and the Great Plague of 1665. It was feared throughout the century, all the more terrifying because its attacks seemed arbitrary. Various treatises on the pestilence were written, many emphasising the spiritual 'wrath of God' aspect. At a time when astrology was still respected by many, the appearance of a comet might foretell or even cause the disaster.

In recent times the disease has been diagnosed as bubonic plague, caused by a bacterium, known since 1970 as *Yersina pestis*, formerly as *Pasturella pestis*. This is carried by a small flea, *Xenopsylla cheopsis*, a parasite of the black rat. The rat dies of plague itself, and its infected fleas then bite humans for want of a better food supply, and so pass the bacteria on. The overcrowded, dirty slums of the poorer parts of cities, without any proper sanitation, let alone disposal of rubbish, were ideal for breeding rats, and so these areas suffered the most. But anyone could pick up the infection.

However, a new theory has emerged in the past few years, proposed by Susan Scott, a demographer, and Christopher Duncan, a Professor of Zoology. Their findings are published in *Return of the Black Death: The World's Greatest Serial Killer*.[1] Careful analysis of local records has suggested that the plague was a viral disease, which passed from person to person by droplet infection. Because it had a long incubation period, travellers could infect many people before they showed symptoms themselves.

It has been thought, in any case, that there were different forms of pestilence. Septicaemic plague, for instance, was considered to be a kind of blood poisoning, giving rise to blue-black blotches on the skin, the so-called plague marks. The classic symptoms of plague included extremely painful swellings of the lymph glands, called buboes, hence the name of bubonic plague. The pneumonic variety affected the lungs, and passed from person to person without benefit of fleas. 'Atichoo, atichoo, we all fall down' is supposed to be an allusion to sudden death, not prevented by the sweet smelling herbs and flowers or 'pocket full of posies' that were carried as a prophylactic. If so, the rhyme was retrospective, as it did not appear until 200 years later.[2]

What could be done by these unfortunate people in the past, when the cause of infection was not understood? From the spiritual point of view, public fast days were proclaimed, and sinners were enjoined to repent. However, civic authorities took a pragmatic view that the disease was passed from person to person. From late medieval times quarantine had been imposed on ships suspected of coming from an infected port, and measures were taken by civil authorities to set sick people apart.

In London, during plague outbreaks, the patient might be taken to a pest-house, probably to die in isolation. But if the pest-houses were full, or there were none in the district, the whole household would be quarantined for 40 days once the sickness was known. 'Lord Have Mercy Upon Us' was written, along with a red cross, on the locked doors where people were shut up, and a guard put on the door. No-one was allowed to enter except a doctor (if he would come), or a plague nurse (often an old, illiterate woman more inclined to pilfer than to help), or the searchers of the dead, who were themselves segregated. The doors were unlocked for the removal of corpses, collected on death-carts for burial. At the height of the epidemic funerals were perfunctory, the bodies tipped hastily into plague pits at night.

People still alive inside the house were dependent on the watchmen for a supply of food and water, which might or might not be supplied. Conditions rapidly became terrible, as can be imagined. Sometimes whole families were found dead together. The practice was justified (by the authorities) as a measure to prevent the spread of infection, but it was frequently a death sentence for those who were healthy to begin with. No wonder, if Scott and Duncan are correct, and the plague was in fact spread by droplet infection. It is not surprising that people tried to conceal the fact of plague in their households, or that remedies were so varied and sometimes bizarre.

Other public health measures were recommended. In 1630, the College of Physicians had suggested that plague was caused by several possible factors, such as overcrowded housing, too many people buried inside churches, including former victims, the sale of meat and fish unfit to eat, low standards of cleanliness in public streets and ditches, stagnant water, rubbish tips (laystalls) close to the city, and slaughterhouses inside it.[3] The King's Physician, Sir Theodore de Mayerne, broadly agreed with all this, adding the movement of vagrants and assembly of people in taverns and alehouses as ways in which the disease was spread. Interestingly, he thought that animals might be implicated too – but advised that cats and dogs should be killed, as well as rats, mice and weasels.

In the household books, there are many receipts for avoidance and treatment, but the disease is not mentioned with more horror than other afflictions. In general, a hopeful note is maintained, though the possibility of death is mentioned.

Early on, the practical Mrs Corlyon devoted a whole chapter of twelve receipts to the problems of plague.[4] This was in 1606, when the outbreak of 1603 must have been fresh in memory. She starts with prevention:

An order of Dyett to be vsed in tyme of Sicknesse and will
preserue the Obseruers thereof from the Plauge [sic][5]
In the morninge at your vprysinge before you do take the ayre burne
Tarre vpon a chafing dishe of cooles, and take the ayre thereof, then
drinck a good draughte of Beere or Ale wherein these hearbes have
stoode all nighte that is to saye) Sage woorme-woode. Hearbegrace

and Plantyn and so soone as you haue dronck out the drincke fyll vpp your pott againe. It is not amiss if you drinck thereof againe in the afternoones and shifte the hearbes twice or thrice a weeke. If you do vse this order and in this sorte in the tyme of infection you shalbe free.

This combines two of the recurring motifs of plague treatments in most collections: a fumigating smell, as of tar, and herbal prophylactics, especially rue. Another suggestion was for a pomander made from melted yellow wax, tar and vinegar, with wormwood powder to make a thick mix. This was made into balls, pierced so that a string could be threaded through and hung round the neck.[6] You could also chew angelica root, orange or lemon peel, or sorrel leaf. She suggests, as well, eating a fig stuffed with rue and walnut, a receipt which recurs many times elsewhere.

Another of her medicines makes a very ambitious claim – that if you take it nine times you are safe for a whole year. A bit of number magic seems to be creeping in here:

A Medecine preseruatiue against the Plague[7]
Take an handfull of Elder leaues an handfull of redd Bramble leaues as much of Herbe Grace [rue], and as much of Sage leaves Washe them and swinge them togeather in a fayre clothe and straine them with a quart of White Wine, and then putt it in a glasse and put to it a good quantitye of Ginger, and drincke a good spoonfull of it, and it shall preserue from the infection for twentye dayes, and nyne times taken shalbe sufficient for a whole yeare.

If, however, in spite of these precautions you did go down with plague, there were three medicines to make you sweat it out, or reduce heat if you became too feverish. One was 'An Almonde milke to coole those that be in the extreeme heate of the Plauge [sic]' Several elaborate medicines of powdered herbs and syrup or honey could be administered too.

The appearance of buboes might be taken as a bad or good sign – bad because they showed how ill the patient was, but good if they broke and subsequently dried up. A poultice of a hot onion could be applied, or if preferred you could combine poultice with prognosis:

A Medecine to trye whether those will live or dye that haue the
Plauge come out vppon them[8]

Take of Gumm called Galbanum and dissolue it with the iuyce
of feilde Dasyes, then spreade it vppon the fleshe syde of Glouers
Leather, but lett the Plaister be no broder then the soore is discollared
then lay it vppon the soore, and holde it on with your hand the
space of a quarter of an hower, and if then it do cleaue [stick on],
the Partye will live without all doubte, if not he will dye. And if it
doe cleaue, it will rypen the Soore, and breake it in 24 howers, and
that before it do come of[f]. Probatum est.

Markham, some years later, has suggestions like Mrs Corylon's for
avoidance and treatment. For instance, you could take his preservative medicine and then 'chaw in your mouth the dried root of
angelica, or smell, as on a nose-gay, to the tasseld end of a ship
rope, and they will surely preserue you from infection.'[9] The idea
that disease was spread by bad smells was widespread, so the end of
a ship's rope, which would probably smell of tar (tar again), would
counteract noxious vapours.

Pepys echoes this, too. On 7 June 1665, he first saw houses marked
with a red cross showing the presence of plague within:[10]

> It put me into an ill conception of myself and my smell [that is,
> what he could smell], so that I was forced to buy some roll-tobacco
> to smell to and chaw, which took away the apprehension.

Houses were frequently scented anyway as part of the good housewife's routine, as for example with 'An excellent sweet water for
a casting bottle'[11] by Sir Hugh Plat, containing oils of lavender,
thyme, lemons, cloves and a little civet. But another stronger
vapour was used for fumigation of houses after plague. Brimstone
was used with or without other spices. You would have needed
a good casting bottle or perfume pot after that to get rid of the
stink of sulphur.

Jane Parker has a simple and reassuring precaution like
Mrs Corlyon's above:

a preservative for the plague[12]
take rew and the kernell of a walnut and bay salt and put it into a
figg and eate it in a morning fasting.

This association of rue, walnut and fig has a very long history indeed.
Dioscorides had claimed that walnuts were an antidote to poison
when eaten with figs and rue. William Turner cites Dioscorides as
one of his authorities for his *Herbal* of 1567, where he repeats the
same assertion. In particular rue, or herb of grace, had an unassaila-
ble reputation as an antidote to poisons and animal venoms. Among
Gerarde's extensive entries for the plant[13] he too quotes a claim of
Dioscorides, that the seeds drunk in wine are:

> ... a counter poyson against deadly medicines, or the poyson of
> Wolfesbane, birdlime, Mushroms or Toadstoole, the bitings of ser-
> pents, stinging of scorpions, spiders; bees, hornets, or waspes, and
> is reported, that if a man be annointed with the iuice of Rue, these
> will not hurt him; and that the serpent is driuen away at the smell
> thereof when it is burned ...

Furthermore, when a weasel has to fight a serpent it eats some rue
before setting out! (Obviously a most useful herb.) But at some
point the general antidote to poison had become a prophylactic
against plague. He continues:

> The leaves of Rue eaten with the Kernels of Walnuts, or figs
> stamped togither and made into a masse or paaste, is good against
> all euill aires, the pestilence or plague, resisteth poison and al
> venom ...

He goes on to quote the Latin poem by Macer, linking rue with
King Mithridates, who used to eat twenty of the leaves with salt
before breakfast to make himself immune to poisons. In this way
it is connected with the medicine Mithridate, described on p. 53.

A very similar receipt, but using thirty or forty rue leaves and
several walnuts, appears in Barrett[14], so the idea was evidently very
popular and continued in use through the century. On leaving

London during the Great Plague, the Auditor of the Exchequer instructed his clerk, who remained behind:

> Lett everyone take every morning a little London Treacle, or the kernell of a walnutt, with five leaves of rue and a grayne of salt beaten together and rosted in a figg, and soe eaten; and never stirre out fasting.[15]

A different prophylactic was recommended by John Allin, who had been deprived of his living as a clergyman because he could not deny the Covenant. He took to the study of medicine and was also an alchemist. He wrote to a friend in 1665:

> ... get a piece of angell gold, if you can of Eliz. coine (that is ye best) which is phylosophicall gold, and keepe it allways in your mouth when you walke out or any sicke persons come to you ... [16]

Philosophical gold was the gold of an Adept, transmuted from base metal. As the Elixir which was said to perform this wonder also had the power of curing disease, it made sense to assume the transmuted gold also had protective or curative properties.

There were persistent stories that alchemical gold had been produced in Elizabethan times. Thomas Charnock claimed to have done so in 1574,[17] and Edward Kelley, who became the associate of Dr John Dee, demonstrated transmutation using a powder found in a Welsh bishop's tomb.[18] However, neither Kelley nor Dee were able to make more of the powder for themselves.

Another theory of the cause and cure of plague went back, of course, to Galen. If it was agreed that disease was caused by putrefaction of humours, you could take a herbal medicine of feverfew, scabious and mugwort 'and it wil expel the corruption'.[19]

Two Plague-Waters were among Sir Kenelm Digby's recipes, collected after his death by his assistant George Hartman, and published in 1669. They are both distillations of herbs in white wine, one slightly more elaborate than the other. The simpler one contains equal weights of rue, rosemary, sage, sorrel, celandine, mugwort, red bramble tops, pimpernel, wild-dragons (a herb), agrimony, balm and angelica, all steeped in the wine for four days and then distilled.[20]

Sometimes, a living creature – or one just killed – was held to the plague sore to draw out its poison. Thus, Markham kept the patient warm in bed until 'the sore beginne to rise; then to the same apply a liue Pidgeon cut in two parts' (though there was an alternative of a poultice).[21]

Jane Parker has this spectacular receipt. The queen mentioned was Henrietta Maria:

> a medison that the Lord maier had from the queen which is a most
> pretious medison for the plague and much aproued[22]
> take a handfull of Sage elder leaues red bramble leaues stampe and
> strayne them together through a cloath with a quart of white wine
> then take a quantity of white wine vinegar and mingle altogether
> and drinke thereof in a morning a sponfull 9 days together and you
> shalbe whole amongst all the excellent medisens for the plague ther
> is none more worthy and aualable then this and when the sore doth
> apeare then take a cocke chickin or a pullet and set the rumpe to the
> sore and let it gape and labour for life and dye and so take another
> and so a thirde keeping the rumpe at the sore tell all the pyson be
> drawn out and the last chicken will live when the venum is out and
> the sore aswage and the party will recouer

The thinking here definitely seems to be that the poison or venom of the sickness will be magically transferred to the unlucky chickens. There is a very similar receipt in *The Queen's Closet Opened* of 1655.[23]

Were such remedies really used? Quite apart from the cruelty involved to the chickens – which probably didn't worry the seventeenth-century plague victim too much – there would be considerable difficulty in keeping a struggling bird applied to a bubo in groin or armpit while one lay seriously ill in bed. But there is a remark by Pepys dated 19 October 1663. Charles II's queen was ill, he writes, 'so ill as to be shaved and pidgeons put to her feet, and to have the extreme unction given her by the priests …' So perhaps this kind of magic did work, for some. The queen recovered from the spotted fever, but we aren't told about the pigeons. Maybe they were half-pigeons, applied for their heat, as birds have a higher temperature than humans.

The following remedies, also from Parker, could have been more practical in an ordinary household:[24]

> for a plague sore
> take the yolke of an egge and turpentine hony and flower of each as much in quantity as the yolke of an egge 6 fleakes of saffron beate this and mingle them well to geather and make them into a salue without fire and this will clense the sore

> to breake the sore
> add to it halfe a lily roote rosted and halfe an oynion rosted as much boter [butter] as a nutmuge and renew it once in 24 houers

FRENCH, ENGLISH OR SPANISH POX

English people referred to it as French, French people called it the English Disease. It could also be attributed to the Spanish. We call it syphilis now. Nobody wanted to claim it, and no wonder, as it was one of the most distressing diseases that it was possible to contract. Not only was the patient ill, but there was a strong element of shame attached to it, as it was known to be associated with sex, especially illicit sex. In the past it was easy to regard it as a punishment for lechery.

We know now that a corkscrew-shaped spirochete, *Treponema pallidum* is to blame. It spread through Europe from the end of the fifteenth century onwards, popularly supposed to have been brought back from the Americas by Christopher Columbus's sailors. Another theory suggests that it had been present in Europe before this, but became especially virulent at this time. Wherever it came from it was feared and hated, and kept secret as much as possible.

One of the nastiest features of the untreated disease is that after its first appearance as a small sore near the site of infection, which apparently heals, there is an interval until the appearance of a rash and other symptoms. This second stage may last for several months, before it too disappears. The third stage may emerge many years later and can lead to a variety of unpleasant forms of death, including insanity caused by lesions in the brain. Those who underwent some form of treatment could therefore think themselves cured because their symptoms had gone. Yet even in the latent periods, the patient was infectious, able to pass on the disease to other innocent people, or to an unborn child, who would then either abort or come into the world with congenital syphilis, failing to thrive and often dying young.

Lady Grace Mildmay is overconfident about her remedy, 'The cure of the pox, the surest, shortest and easiest that ever was found.'[25] She started by bleeding the sufferer, who was kept on a light diet for a fortnight and dosed with a herbal purge. Then came rubbing with a distilled lotion of sublimate of mercury, arsenic, several herbs, aqua vitae and rose water. The patient was kept wrapped up except for the part being rubbed, and there was 'a great fire in the chamber' to keep warm by. Then the person went to bed, covered liberally with bedclothes to induce sweating, with the fire kept going night and day. He was not allowed out of bed, even to feed, but 'his drink being as whole as may be.' He must have needed a lot of liquid. 'The patient must sweat as long as ever he is able to endure and when he hath sweated enough, he must be dried and shifted, keeping the sheet and shirt for once or twice more at the most. The sweating being done without taking any air, all the while.'

Markham too uses an ointment of quicksilver, that is mercury, 'and kill it with fasting spittle', plus verdigris, gum arabic, turpentine, olive oil and poplar bud ointment to rub onto the sores, '& keepe the party exceeding warme.'[26] Saliva, especially that of a person who was fasting, had been thought to be curative at least as far back as Pliny.[27]

Mrs Corlyon has 'A Medecine to cure a face that is Redd and full of Pimples',[28] which is so similar that I suspect it was a tactful way of alluding to the pox. It starts with two pennyworth of quicksilver, slaked again with 'fasting spittle'. It was then ground up with oil of bay, and tempered with woodbine water. This was used to anoint the face morning and evening for fourteen days 'keeping your selfe close in your chamber all that tyme.'

Starting a week before this treatment, during the anointing period and for a week afterwards, the patient had to drink beer with the addition of half a pound of madder to ten gallons, which was then allowed to go stale. Madder is better known as a dye than as a medicine, but Culpeper says that it is useful to remove urinary gravel, against palsy, sciatica and bruises. Applied externally it clears up freckles, 'morphew and white scurf, or any such deformity of the skin' so there is a link with the red pimples.

Mrs Corlyon's patient is warned that the face will look worse than before for a week after treatment, 'vntill such tyme as the humor be killed, that is betwixte the fleshe and the skinn.'

Mercury is itself poisonous, so the pox victim was in an unenviable position. Nevertheless, mercury continued to be used until the advent of Salvarsan, based on arsenic, at the beginning of the twentieth century.[29]

Guaiacum wood, imported from the West Indies and South America by the Spanish, and the enterprising Fuggers, had been an alternative treatment for the French pox in Elizabethan times, but it had fallen into disrepute by the seventeenth century. It was attacked by Paracelsus (as were strong preparations of mercury), but still appears in Culpeper's translation of the 1618 *Pharmacopoeia Londinensis*:[30]

> *Guajacum, Lignum vitae.* Dries, attenuates causeth sweat, resisteth putrifaction, is admirable good for the French pocks, as also for Ulcers, Scabs and Leprosie.

With the sweating, which was also induced by mercury, we are back with the idea of expelling sickness by evacuation.

SMALLPOX

The disease was widespread, affecting all social classes. King Charles II's younger brother, the Duke of Gloucester, died from it soon after the Restoration. John Evelyn lost two daughters to it. Queen Mary, of the William-and-Mary duo, died of it in 1694. However, it was not invariably fatal, but survivors were usually left with scars or pock-marks, a serious matter for girls who needed husbands, as most did. The household books have more receipts for minimising, healing or covering up these scars than for treating the illness in the first place (see p. 169).

Hannah Woolley is moderately dismissive, comparing it with measles, though measles could also be dangerous. The important thing was to prevent a child 'murdering' her complexion by scratching in either case:

> *What is best to be administred to one sick of the Measels*[31]
> In this distemper, as in the small Pox, it is only necessary to defend the Heart, and preserve the Stomach, from putrefaction, and corruption: if young, to hinder the hands from murdering a good face: and then give the diseased a Julip, made of two ounces of Violets, four ounces of Rose-water, and four grains of Oyl of Vitriol, mix them and let them be drunk cold. It is as good a receipt as any for this distemper.

It might be thought that sulphuric acid – oil of vitriol – would do little to preserve the stomach, even in small quantities.

Consumption (Tuberculosis)

This was another killer. In the plague year of 1665, there were also nearly 5,000 deaths from consumption in London. In the previous year, Pepys' brother had succumbed to it. So, too, ten years previously, had Nicholas Culpeper, in spite of all his knowledge of physick, dying at the age of thirty-seven.

Ordinary coughs and colds were treated with a mixture of herbs, very commonly including horehound and liquorice. Here is an example from *The Queens Closet*:

> A drink for cold Rhumes and Flegms.[32]
> Take the roots of Fennel, Comfrey, Parsley and Liverwort, Heartstongue [sic] Mousear, Horehound, Sandrake, Maiden-hair, Cinquefoyl, Hysop, Bugloss and Violet leaves of each one handful,

wash and dry them very clean, Raysins solis eight ounces, Aniseeds four drams, Liquorish two drams, Elecampane roots two drams, half a pinte of Barley washed and bruised, boyl these in a pottle [half a gallon] of fair water, until half the liquor be consumed, strain it, and put to it one quart of white or Rhenish Wine, and one ounce of Sugarcandy, and boyl it again till half be consumed, take it from the fire, and when it is cold put it into a clean glass, and drink thereof every morning and evening a draught first and last, and by Gods grace it will make you well and sound. *Approved*

There is a theme in all these – in modern terms they are expectorants, soothing to throat, diuretic, anti-inflammatory, antiseptic, good for catarrh, good for respiratory infections and chronic bronchitis. Even with half the herbs, this is a cough medicine which would probably have worked.

But consumption was a much more serious matter. Treatments varied from the sensible, building up the patient with milk and eggs for instance, to the exotic, such as the use of dried and powdered foxes' lungs.[33]

The Renaissance magical philosophy of Cornelius Agrippa taught that an excess of any property in something provoked a similar property elsewhere. Thus fire led to fire, and water to water. He said that doctors used brains to treat brains, and lungs to help lung disease.[34] The tradition went back even before the Renaissance. Dioscorides had used them as a remedy for asthma. Foxes' lungs, well dried, were included in Culpeper's *Physical Directory* as 'an admirable strengthener of the lungues.'[35] The magic meant that a healthy animal's lungs could restore those of a human being.

Mrs Corlyon has many receipts for chest complaints, including consumption. Of course it was better not to 'fall into' the disease in the first place:

A speciall good Medicine and will keepe those that doe vse to take it from falling into a Consumption[36]

Take two new laid Egges and sett them in the embers vntill they be thorowghe warme, but lett not the white be harde, then make litle hooles in the toppes of them and poure out the whites as cleane as you

can and fyll vpp your egges with redd Rose water; and the powder
of Cynamome and Sugar, then warme them againe in the embers and
so eate them. Vse this and you shall fynde it very effectual.

Her 'Medicine for one that is in a Consumption' is along the same
lines, but is basically an egg custard made with cow's or goat's milk
and the yolk of a poached egg, sweetened. Another was a distilled
water made with a pint of new milk, a pint of red rose water, the
yolks of thirty new-laid eggs and an ounce of bruised cinnamon.
I doubt if much more than cinnamon-and-rose flavoured water
would have emerged.

Another interesting ingredient frequently included in cough and
chest medicines was snails. This short receipt from the collection of
Mrs Miller includes calves' lung and snails, distilled in a cold still:

Calves Lung water for a consumption[37]
One gallon of milk, The lungs of a calf whilst warm cut in pieces,
a peck of garden snails, bruise them till the shells are broke, twelve
whites of Eggs, four Nutmegs sliced, Distill these all together in a
cold still, stir it sometimes in distilling. You may drink from one
quart a day to two quarts, warm it milk warm when you drink it
and sweeten it to your Taste with white sugar=candy or loaf sugar.
Mrs Sutton

Dr Gideon Harvey disapproved of distillation of snails. Here is his
reasoning, and an explanation of why snails were used at all:

The Description of Aqua Limacum Magistralis, *or the* London Snail
Water, *against Consumption*[38]
This compound Water is so ridiculous, that I am ashamed to see it
in any *Dispensatory*; for the chief thing aimed at is, through the cool
clammy and glutinous substance of the Liquor of the Snails, 1. To
cool the heat of the Hectick Fever. 2. To repair the parts consumed.
3. To facilitate Expectoration, that is, to make the matter come up
easie by cough, through its lenifying [softening] quality, whereby it
sweeteneth the humors, by allaying those gnawing Salts, that prey
on the Lungs. Now in distilling of the Snails, there is no part of

> their unctuous or glutinous Liquor passeth the Alembick, but a meer Elementary Water ...

Instead, he recommended a liquor of well-washed garden snails, with the addition of ground ivy, speedwell, lungwort, scabious, burnet, coltsfoot and nettletops, liquorice, stoned dates, marshmallow seeds, saffron and the 'greater cold seeds': cold according to Galenic principles, that is '1. Pompion. 2. Cucumber. 3. Gourge. 4. Melon Seeds.'

All these were put with spring water into a sealed pipkin and heated in a large pan of water for twelve hours. Then the liquid was strained and sweetened with honey, 'put it into a glass, and keep it in the Cellar.'

Nourishing broths, especially containing china root, were a way of treating the wasting disease, but nevertheless it must have been agonising to witness someone dwindling away towards death. Sometimes, desperation called for magic and expense to be incorporated into the soup. A receipt from the Barrett manuscript, quoted in full on p. 196, is one such. It is a 'raire watter' distilled from a cock, half a gallon of sack, milk, dried fruit, herbs, rose water, hartshorn and china root – plus sugar candy, gold, musk, ambergris, horn of unicorn and bezoar stone. Very expensive, but when a life was obviously ebbing it may have helped to realise how much one was prized by the family who were paying for these costly ingredients. As far as the family was concerned, too, perhaps they felt that they had done their utmost for the patient.

7

Diet, Digestion and Food as Medicine

Food was an important part of the regimen described by Galen. Following him, the classical medicine of the physicians laid emphasis on general lifestyle. A good and healthy life was based on six so-called 'non-naturals', which were wholesome air, food and drink, sleep and waking, movement and rest, retaining and evacuation, and control of emotion. The air was to be healthy (we would say non-polluted), food and drink suitable for the individual, sufficient, but not too much, hours of slumber and alertness balanced, with neither excessive. The body should retain what was taken in to extract its goodness, but then evacuate the residue, and sex was included in evacuation. Emotional wellbeing was also important. Who could quarrel with such ideals? They are as important today as they ever were in the past. But, unfortunately, accidents, infections, famine, madness, war, poverty and oppression sometimes get in the way of the ideal.

DIET

In the seventeenth century, recipes for cooking were important, but advice on what we would consider a good diet was scanty. Copies of Andrew Boorde's *A Compendyous Regyment or A Dyetary of Helth*[1] might still be taken down from dusty bookshelves. Boorde had been a monk, but was released from his vows. He travelled extensively and wrote a traveller's guide to Europe, as well as practising medicine and producing this entertaining handbook on diet and health, based on Galenic principles. For example, various kinds of flesh had good and bad properties:

> Of all tame fowle a capon is moste beste, For it is nutrytyue, and is soone dygestyd … The flesshe of a cocke is harde of dygestyon, but the broth or gely made of a cocke is restoratyue. pygyons be good for coloryke & melancoly men. … [2]
> Beefe is a good meate for an Englysshe man, so be it the beest be yonge, & that it be not kowe-flesshe; For olde beefe and kowe flesshe doth ingender melancolye and leporouse humoures.[3]

Near the beginning of the seventeenth century, an educated person could appreciate Sir John Harington's translation into English of the *Regimen Sanitatis Salerni*. This originally medieval work gave mainly Hippocratic rules for health. Good advice sometimes, such as to avoid stress, keep cheerful and eat properly:

> Use three Physicions still; First Doctor *Quiet*,
> Next Doctor *Merry-man*, and Doctor *Dyet*.[4]

It was not always helpful about individual foods, though. Figs, for instance, were all right for external application, but eating them was not a good idea (unless to prevent plague, as already described). 'By Figges are lice ingendred, Lust provoken.' A basket of figs was a classical symbol of fertility[5] so the association with lust was understandable, but where did the lice come from? Possibly they were small maggots. The idea that some creatures could arise from rotten matter was not disproved until the eighteenth century. Some insects have almost invisibly small eggs, so until microscopes were used scientifically it looked as if vermin could emerge spontaneously.

Prejudice against other fresh fruit is apparent as well. Cold and moist foods encouraged phlegm:

> By Nuts, Oyle, Eeles, and cold in head,
> By Apples and raw fruits is hoarsenesse bred.

Yet the herbals sometimes gave indications of the qualities of hot, cold, moist and dry of some foods, so that a hot fever could be balanced by cooling fruits for instance. Here for example is Culpeper on strawberries:[6]

> ... The fruit when green, is cool and dry; but when ripe cool and moist; the berries cool the liver, the blood and the spleen, or a hot choleric stomach ...

However, by the mid-seventeenth century, there seems to have been less conviction about what formed a proper diet. Poorer people could never pick and choose, in any case. Markham praised 'the excellency of Oates' partly because they were cheap, partly because they were nutritious for man and beast.[7] At the end of the century John Evelyn extolled fruit and vegetables, arguing indeed in favour of a frugal vegetarian or near vegetarian diet, with many appeals to classical and biblical precedents. He was a member of The Royal Society, and dedicated his book on salads, *Acetaria*, to its President.

It is difficult, of course, to judge exactly how much fresh food was in fact consumed, as no written recipe is needed to pick and munch an apple from the tree, for instance. There are certainly some receipts for sallets (salads) in most cookery collections. Even the *Forme of Cury* has one. Markham has many, some raw, served with oil, vinegar and seasoning, and some of cooked or pickled vegetables. Some were 'for shewe only' as a table decoration.[8] There are plenty of recipes in cookery collections for fruit pies, tarts, conserves and pickles, but few by comparison mention fresh fruit. For instance, in Hannah Woolley's *Bill of Fare of suitable Meat for every Month in the Year*,[9] you could have 'Straw berries and Cream. Or Straw-berries, White-wine, Rosewater and Sugar' in June, and 'Some Creams and Fruit' in August and September, otherwise warden pears, gooseberries, codling apples and quinces are cooked in tarts or pies.

Occasionally, a reader of receipt books is warned to avoid more specific foodstuffs, such as too much sugar:

> ...the immoderate use thereof is dangerous, for it will rot the Teeth, and taint the Breath, ingender Jaundies and Consumptions ... [10]

SCURVY

The fact that there are many receipts purporting to cure scurvy show that it was probably widespread, an indication of poor diet. Full-blown scurvy only appears after an absence of Vitamin C for several *months!*

Gerarde missed a breakthrough by a single concept. If he had realised that scurvy was a disease not caused *by* something in the diet, but by a *lack* of something, he might have become the patron saint of seafarers. He knew how to cure the condition. Writing of spoonwort, or scurvy grass, he says the juice, given in ale or beer, 'is a singular medicine against ... the disease called ... in English the Scuruie.' It was a deadful thing:

> The gums are loosed, swolne and exulcerate; the mouth greeuously stinking; the thighes and legs are withall verie often full of blewe spots, not much unlike those that come of bruses: the face and the rest of the bodie is oftentimes of a pale colour; and the feete are swolne, as in the dropsie.[II]

He knew where it was likely to break out, but made erroneous, though reasonable, guesses as to causes:

> ... a disease haunting the campes, which vex them there that are besieged and pinned vp: and it seemeth to come by eating of salt meates, which is increased and cherished with the colde vapours of the stone wals ... [also] much sleepe and rest on shipboorde ...

(Would the average seaman, working a sailing ship in all tides and weathers, have agreed he had too much sleep and rest?) But Gerarde recommended ships' surgeons to carry the juice of scurvy-grass in a bottle with a narrow neck, with oil on top to stop it putrefying.

In the household books, scurvy grass, brooklime and other anti-scorbutic herbs come up many times, but all too often they are boiled or otherwise heated, which would have destroyed most of the vitamin C they contain. Mrs Corlyon's book has a receipt which contains plenty of good herbs, but they are thoroughly boiled and the water used to bathe the afflicted legs! There is another which comes much closer to a cure, with many handfuls of herbs put into a bag and soaked in ale, *not* heated.[12] They included watercress, brooklime, rosemary and scurvy grass, as well as others. *The Queen's Closet* has a similar receipt, attributed to the Countess of Arundel.[13] This lady owned a copy of Mrs Corlyon's manuscript, so it may have been adapted from the earlier one. A later receipt in *The Queen's Closet* uses watercress, brooklime and (hurrah!) oranges and juice of scurvy grass, but (alas!) reverts to boiling them again – yet adds (hurrah!), when cold, 'three or four Limons more …' It might have been, as it claimed, 'very good for them that have the Scurvy, or are inclined to it.'

Enlightenment was coming, but too slowly for general improvement in this century. (It was not until 1795 that citrus juice was issued to sailors in the British Navy.) John Evelyn's *Acetaria* is partly a list of food plants, partly a celebration of preparing and eating them, and partly a philosophical work about the best food for mankind. He had made practical observations though:

> … it seem in general, that raw *Sallets* and *Herbs* have experimentally been found to be the most soveraign Diet in that *Endemial* (and indeed with us, *Epidemical* and almost universal) Contagion the *Scorbute* [scurvy] … [14]

Not much, perhaps, but an enquiry that would later bear fruit in several senses.

DIGESTIVE DISTURBANCES

The process of digestion was seen as a kind of cooking in the stomach. It was frequently a painful, windy process. Many receipts for the relief of colic are based on spices such as aniseed, cumin, caraway and fennel, still used to ease digestion. Sometimes, the medicines double for the relief of stone or gravel. Mrs Corlyon has a lot of suggestions. This one might cure rumblings due to hunger, too:

A Medecine for winde in the Stomake[15]
Take a new laid Egg and roste it reare then open the topp of it and

putt out the white that lyeth on the toppe then temper your egge
with a good quantity of Pepper and Annysseedes brused and so eate
it fasting, and in the after noone if there be greate cause continue
thus a good space and it will helpe

There was occasionally a mixture of spices and so on which one would
expect to be taken internally – but no, it had a different application.
For instance 'A very good Medecine to putt away any greefe from
the Stomake or to disgest a Surfett'[16] consists of a thick piece of toast
soaked with aquavitae or Malmsey, sprinkled with powder of mint
and wormwood, cloves, mace and a little nutmeg. It was then put on
the stomach as hot as was bearable, bandaged in place, left for twelve
hours, 'and then renewe it or change it at your discretion. This do
as often as you shall see cause.' It is as if the spices could be absorbed
through the skin or navel. Probably the warmth helped.

A peculiar receipt from *The Queen's Closet* puts a cold weight on
the stomach, which probably wouldn't have done much good:

The Lady Drury's Medicine for the Colick proved[17]
Take a turf of green Grass, and lay it to the Navil, and let it lye till
you finde ease, the green side must be laid next to the Belly.

It might be a half-remembered version of a receipt which Mrs
Corlyon used for a stitch in the side.[18] She had taken a slice of
well-compacted earth from a floor, sprinkled it with vinegar and
heated it on a gridiron. Then it was wrapped in a linen cloth and
applied to the area of pain. This would have been quite a good
poultice which would have retained heat for a long time.

Acid indigestion might be helped by the Kidders' remedy:

A present remedy for the grips or flux of the guts[19]
Take allybaster and burn it in the fier and then scrape it into milke
and boyle it then let the party Drink of it when he pleases

You might tackle the problem from a reverse position, too, with a
glister (an enema) or a suppository, which might also be used for constipation. 'A Suppositer good for those that ar troubled with the Collicke

or winde'[20] consisted of half a flattened fig, with some bay salt rolled
up inside it, skin inwards. This was then tied with thread to make it
slightly conical, greased with butter, and so 'ministered' to the patient.

Lax, flux, or worse, the bloody flux troubled many. Severe diarrhoea can kill, especially children, through dehydration. It can be
caused by many conditions, some serious, such as typhoid fever and
dysentery, some not, such as the 'tummy bugs' that still occur. Food
poisoning spread by flies and unwashed hands, suspect water supplies,
food going off in warm weather – the housewife had ample reasons
to consult her book if she had one, or to compile one if she had not.

Mrs Corlyon, of course, had a number of helpful suggestions for
the bloody flux.[21] She has various internal medicines of herbs, or
eggs, medicinal almond milk, a concentrated broth of chicken taken
half an hour before meals, 'drinck smale drinck and alwayes put a
gadd of steele redd hott into the same', like heating punch with a hot
poker. You should lie down to rest for an hour in the afternoon, 'and
binde your armes aboue your ellbowes as hard as you can suffer it for
the space of an hower, and stirr litle be quiett and merrye.' Relaxing
would be fine, but why a tight band above the elbows should help,
she does not explain. The list goes on, including a syrup of the
four (Galenic) cold seeds from the apothecary's with woodbine and
plantain water, 'This will purge the blood'. According to this lady
the cold seeds were those of 'Cowecumbers, Millions, Pompions
and Gourdes', and the four lesser cold seeds were 'Lettice Parselyne
Endeeue and Succhorye.'[22]

A separate receipt uses an unexpected ingredient:

An approued Medecine for the stoppinge of a fluxxe[23]
Take a good quantity of Sea Cooles beyinge beaten as fyne to powder
as you can, put it into Beere or Ale mingle and stirr it well and let
the Patient drinck thereof. And if he cannot take the powder in that
sorte, lett it stand all nighte, and straine the drincke in the morninge,
and let the Patient vse it at all tymes when he drincketh for the space
of 2. or 3. dayes and by Gods helpe it will cure.

Sea coal was coal mined in the Newcastle area, brought south by
ship down the east coast, and normally used as fuel. The coal was

tarry and sulphurous, causing an unpleasant smoke, so just possibly some of the tar might be dissolved in the beer, and disinfect the gut – but I wouldn't like to try it myself.

The opposite of flux was costiveness, caused perhaps by the comparative lack of fruit and vegetables in the diet. A gentle laxative was required. The Townsend manuscript has 'A purging broth yet Comfortable'.[24] It was beef broth with raisins, currants, fennel and other flavouring herbs, liverwort and scabious, plus half an ounce of the best senna. Senna is mentioned again and again as an effective laxative, still to be found in our bathroom cabinets. It could be bruised and put into a linen bag, for instance, with polypodium of the oak, bayberries, aniseeds and fennel seeds also bruised, plus a stone to make it sink, then dropped into new ale to soak for a week.[25] One hopes that it was carefully labelled, too.

The Parker manuscript has a receipt for 'purging prunes to purge gently 6 or 7 times'.[26] (Prunes are favourite for breakfast even today.) They 'worke soe gently that if the weather be warme the patien need not keepe his chamber.' You could not risk going too far from your close-stool or privy if you had taken a strong purge. Pepys spent a Sunday in February 1661 in seclusion 'took physique all day, and God forgive me, did spend it in reading of some little French romances.'[27]

Purging was done not only to relieve constipation, but as a preliminary to various treatments, to rid the body of excess humours, or as spring-cleaning. Culpeper gives general advice on purging in his *Directions* which introduce his *Physical Directory*. For example, one should 'Consider what the humor offending is, and let the Medicine be such as purgeth that humor, else you will weaken nature, not the disease.' Later he says:

> But all violent purges require a due ordering of the body, such ought to be taken in the morning after you are up, and not to sleep after them, before they have done working, at least before night, two hours after you have taken them, drink a draught of warm posset drink or broath, and six hours after, eat a bit of Mutton, often walking about the chamber, let there be a good fire in the chamber, and stir not out of the camber [sic] till the purge have done working, or not till next day.[28]

Glisters were enemas, administered with enthusiasm. They, too, served different, and one might think, opposite purposes. Mrs Corlyon had one for the colic,[29] another for the bloody flux,[30] made of fresh warm cow's milk, mutton or goat's fat and sugar. But one would have thought that glisters (or clisters) were best for the relief of constipation, as Hannah Woolley says:

> A very safe Clister to be used by either Man or Woman who is much bound or costiv.[31]

> Take Mallows and Mercury [the herb] unwasht, of each two handfuls, half an handful of Barley; clean rubbed and washed, and boil them in Spring-water, from a pottle [half a gallon] to a quart, then strain out the Water, and put it in a Skillet, and put to it three spoonfuls of Sallet-oyl, two spoonfuls of Honey and a little Salt, then make it luke-warm, and with your Pipe administer it.

Emetics were given, like some purges, to get rid of the wrong kind of humour. They could be comparatively mild, as Gerarde's mixture of vinegar and honey (oxymel) in which horseradish rinds were infused for three days,[32] or violent and dangerous, as he says of stavesacre,[33] which is better used to get rid of vermin, under its other country name of lousewort.

INTESTINAL WORMS

These, like fluxes, were a problem, and could even cause death. The Bill of Mortality for the Plague Year in London had 2,614 fatalities from 'Teeth and Worms', though how many of each is not stated. Many of the household books and herbals have remedies for them. As might be expected, wormwood comes high on the list of cures, but is by no means exclusively for worms, nor the only herb that can be tried. Tansy is also good. Gerarde says 'The seede of the Tansie is a singular and approved medicine against woormes, for in what sort soever it be taken, it killeth and driveth them foorth.'

Hannah Woolley has 'An excellent Water for the Worms'[34] containing wormseed, hartshorn, peach-flowers dried, aloes, and waters of tansy, rue, peach-flowers and wormwood.

One might try more exotic remedies, too:

A great Cordiall to drive out any infection of Worms ./.[35]
Take :4: ounces of unicornes=horne, & as much mithridate as a Beane, & mingle them together, & then dissolve them in two spoons-fulls of white wine, & take it & keep you warme

Magical items such as unicorn's horn appear in the *Pharmacopoeia Londinensis*,[36] though hartshorn is an equivalent. It was said to resist poison, here perhaps, with the mithridate, as an antidote too. There seems to be a sense therefore that worms can be eliminated in the same way as poison.

Even stranger, to us, is the habit of using an ointment, applied externally, though using ingredients known to be effective vermifuges. Mrs Corlyon has internal medicines as well, but how did this one work?

A Medecine for the Wormes eyther in olde Folkes or Children. It will procure loosenesse and is good to prevent an Agewe in a Childe[37] Take an handfull of wormewood and as much of Fetherfewe and fower vnsett Leekes, chopp all these togeather and mingle them with the Gall of a Beeste, then frye them in sweete butter and when they be fryed putt them in the fouldes of a clothe and so lay it to the Stomake, and lett it come ouer the Nauell fasten it and lett it lye two dayes and two nightes and then chaunge it if you see cause.

Perhaps, as in the receipt for wind above, there was a belief that medicine could be absorbed into the stomach via the navel.

OVERINDULGENCES

On occasion, people ate too much for comfort. Mrs Corlyon has 'An excellent water good for a Surfett approued by my self and others'[38] Excellent it may have been, and apparently much needed, as it was made on an industrial scale. Twenty-seven different herbs were gathered, totalling eighty-seven handfuls, with three pounds of aniseeds and two pounds of liquorice. The herbs were dried and then soaked in strong Spanish wine or 'mightye stronge Ale', which was then distilled and kept for use 'when good occasion is offered'.

At the end of the century the Kidders had a far simpler distilled water receipt:

> A very good surphitt watter[39]
> Take sperment cardis [carduus benedictus] & wormod [wormwood] and the newe milke from the cowes and still it with a soft fier you may alsoe doe it in whit wine shred the hearbes small & steep them in the whit wine all night & couer the top of the still with a wet cloth then drye it of sloly [slowly].

Large amounts of wine were imported for the rich and middling sort. Ale and beer was drunk by everyone (very sensibly) in preference to water, and tea and coffee were only just becoming fashionable in the middle of the century. Some drunkenness was probably inevitable. It does not attract much comment in the household books, though Markham does have one helpful receipt:

> Against drunkennes.[40]
> If you would not bee drunke, take the powder of Betany and cole-worts mixt together; and eate it euery morning fasting as much as will lie vpon a sixpence, and it will preserue a man from drunkenness.

Colewort goes back a long way as a preservative from the vine. Both Culpeper and Gerarde say that there is a natural enmity between the two plants, so that one will die where the other grows. Then, there is a leap of magical logic. If colewort (cabbage) will spoil a vine, then it will counteract the effects of wine. It is commended 'being eaten before meat to keep one from surfeiting, as also from being drunk with too much wine, or quickly makes a man sober that is drunk before ...'[41]

If overindulgence had made you fat, there were also a couple of pointers for slimming from Markham. 'For fatnesse and short breath' one should make toasts of unleavened bread, dip them in clarified honey and 'eate this divers times with your meate.'[42] 'For fatnesse about the hart' in the later edition he has a kind of candy made of fennel juice and honey, to be eaten twice a day 'and it wil consume away the fatnesse.' According to Culpeper on fennel 'Both leaves, seeds and roots thereof, are much used in drink or broth, to make people lean that are too fat.'[43] Is it possible that this herb will be our next slimming aid?

FOOD AS MEDICINE: BROTHS

There was less distinction between food and medicine in the seventeenth century than today. Broths, possets, caudles, creams, conserves and cordial waters (see p. 47) were consumed by the healthy as well as the sick. Mrs Corlyon however devotes a whole long chapter to Broths, with twenty-five different receipts, some simply nourishing and easily digestible, others directed to specific conditions. She would have agreed with Dr Boorde that chicken broth was restorative. More than half the receipts in this chapter include chicken, capon or cockerel:

A very comfortable Brothe for any weaknesse[44]
Take to a good bigg Chicken 3. quarts of water and lett it seethe on the fyer keepinge it well scummed. Then take one handfull of Scabious as much of Endeeue, halfe an handfull of Succhory as much of Egremonye as much of Maydenheare a good quantitye of Lyuerwoorte Of Fennell rootes 3. Of Persely rootes as many Of ye-ollow Docke rootes two, and these must be well washed and scraped and the pithe cleane taken out of them. Then take one handfull of Prunes one handfull of Reysons of the Sonn, as many of Currantes and a quantitye of whole Mace euery of these fruytes must be washed very cleane and then putt with the rest into the pott. Lett all stewe togeather a good while and then putt to them the bottome of a Manchett [a small loaf]. Then lett all seeth togeather till the

Brothe begynn to chaunge to a reddish colour, and be not in quantitye past one quart and so straine the same and keepe it. Continue
this Brothe 14. dayes togeather. It must be taken lukewarme once in
the morninge and againe one hower before Supper.

Here for comparison is a standard broth by Gervase Markham:

To make ordinary stewed broth.[45]
To make ordinary stewed broth, you shall take a necke of veale, or
a leg, or marybones of beefe, or a pullet, or mutton, and, after the
meat is washt, put it into a pot with faire water, and being ready
to boile, scumme it well; then you shall take a couple of manchets,
and, paring away the crust, cut it into thicke slices and lay them in a
dish, and couer them with hot broth out of the pot; when they are
steept, put them and some of the broth into a strainer, and straine
it, and then put it into the pot; then take halfe a pound of Prunes,
halfe a pound of Raisins, and a quarter of a pound currants clean
pickt & washed, with a little whole Mace of [sic] and two or three
brused Cloues, and put them into the pot and stirre all well together,
and so let them boile till the meate be enough; then if you will alter
the colour of the broth, put in a little Turnesole or red Saunders
[vegetable colourings] and so serue it vp vpon Sippets, and the fruit
uppermost.

Although there is a strong resemblance between these two dishes,
Mrs Corlyon's receipt had additional herbs. According to Culpeper,
their properties include: scabious, good for coughs, endive, cooling
and cleansing, succory, removed choler and phlegm and was a diuretic, agrimony, cleansing and good for coughs, as was maidenhair,
also a diuretic. Liverwort, as the name implies, was a general tonic
for the liver. Prunes, raisins and currants would be laxative in effect.
The broth was thus an adaptation of a common dish, the herbs
making it to some extent medicinal. It would have been of value
to stimulate appetite.

Others in the broths chapter are for more specific complaints.
For example, this one is for back pain, diarrhoea or diminished
natural spirits. A concentrated chicken broth, where the flesh was

not eaten, but gold added to its value, could be made by very long, gentle heating in a kind of double-boiler. The inner pot was sealed down to prevent evaporation. Someone must have stayed up all night to keep the outer large pan topped up with hot water. The resulting liquid would have been clear, as it was just allowed to run off without pressing:

> A very comfortable receipte for those that haue paine in theire Backes. It will staye the Bodye that is troubled withe any kinde of Fluxx or with the wast of Nature[46]
>
> Take a redd Cocke of a yeare and halfe olde beynge plucked and drawen, chopp hym in peeces and bruse the bones well, then putt hym into a pewter pott of a Pottell [capacity of half a gallon] vn-washed with the bloode feete heade and all and throwe thereone halfe a spoonefull of Salte, putt thereto a pinte of Muscadell halfe a pinte of redd Rose water, 6. Dates cutt in peeces and three or fower Maces Then shake all these well togeather in your pott, you may putt thereto what golde you please more or lesse but the more you doe putt in the more effectually it will worke. Then past downe the couer of your pott, and tye a clothe so close about it that no ayre goe eyther in or out. Sett it into a kettell or pott of seething water vpp to the neck, and lett it so boile contynually the space of 24 howers, and as the water doth wast fyll vpp your kettell againe with hott water, then take out the pott and poure it into a strayner and lett the lyquor run into a Vessell so longe as it will run but wringe it not. Then putt it vpp as you will keepe it. Geue the Patient therof warmed 3. or 4. spoonefulles at a tyme and continue it as you shall see cause, and it will ease you shall haue as much liquor when it is strayned as you did putt into the pott. This is called the distillinge of a Cocke

Mental disturbances, or at least a melancholy humour, could be treated with much the same ingredients. Another receipt is for a literal distillation of a young bird, with milk, rosewater and herbs, not only good for 'those that ar broughte weake with an Agewe or such like Sicknesse', but 'It is very nourishinge and good to putt away Melancholye.'[47]

Sometimes, the broth could be even more concentrated, like this receipt for 'A very comfortable Jellye for those that ar weake'.[48] Two capons, fat removed, were soaked all night then boiled with two gallons of water in a 'very well scoured' pot. The broth was skimmed, the fat taken off, then boiled 'softly a long tyme' until it started to become a 'stiffe Jellye'. The whole lot was strained and cooled before removing all the fat. Then it was re-melted with sugar and salt to taste, plus a spoonful or two of rosewater and vinegar. It was further clarified by having six beaten egg whites added before it boiled, and then strained through a jelly bag containing a sprig of rosemary. After that it was fit for use.

In 1669, sixty-three years after Mrs Corylon's manuscript was produced, there came *The Closet of the Eminently Learned Sir Kenelme Digbie Kt. Opened*. Digby had collected many receipts during his extensive diplomatic travels, and after his death they were fashioned into a book and published by permission of his son. The book was at the aristocratic end of the market. It frequently mentions the Queen, Henrietta Maria, the same Queen whose Closet had been Opened by Mr W. M. in 1655.

Broth was still one of the staples of healthy living. (The learned knight was very fond of mead as well.) He has several receipts for '*Potage de Santé*' or health-soup. One[49] was attributed to the 'very Valetudinary' M. de St. Evremont, a French soldier living in England. As he died aged about 90, perhaps there *was* something in his soup ... It took all the morning to make it, starting at 'nine of the Clock forenoon' when he – or more likely his cook – started to boil a knuckle of veal and a hen. The hen was removed shortly afterwards, then replaced at half past ten with a handful of white endive.

Being careful about his *santé*, the French soldier had to observe the correct balance of 'hot' or 'cold' food according to circumstance. 'When he is in pretty good health, that he may venture upon more savoury hotter things, he puts in a large Onion stuck round with Cloves, and sometimes a little bundle of Thyme and other hot savoury herbs.' These would be taken out and discarded after half an hour's boiling. At eleven thirty, he added two handfuls of tender sorrel, and one each of borage, bugloss, with lettuce and purslane, if available, plus a little chervil and some beet-leaves. At a quarter to twelve some of the broth would be poured over dry bread in a separate dish, with more added as the bread soaked it up, and stewed gently. When the bread was as soft as jelly the dish was filled with broth, the hen and veal put on top and covered with herbs. The soldier had it served up some time after twelve o'clock, but kept part of the broth to drink later, or next morning.

Sometimes a much simpler pick-me-up was needed. Sir Kenelm recommended a nice cup of tea, but with a difference. This recipe derived from a Jesuit from China.[50] Tea was at this time being imported by the East India Company:

> ... To near a pint of the infusion [of tea], take two yolks of new laid-eggs, and beat them very well with as much fine Sugar as is sufficient for this quantity of Liquor; when they are very well incorporated, pour your Tea upon the Eggs and Sugar, and stir them well together. So drink it hot. This is when you come home from attending business abroad, and are very hungry, and yet have not conveniency to eat presently [at once] a competent meal. This presently discusseth and satisfieth all rawness and indigence of the stomack, flyeth suddainly over the whole body and into the veins, and strengthneth exceedingly, and preserves one a good while from necessity of eating.

FOOD AS MEDICINE: POSSETS AND CAUDLES

Possets were drinks made from milk and an acid such as wine to make it curdle, often with eggs and spices added. It has something in common with a medieval caudle, which was a liquid dish made sometimes with almond milk, and included a thickening. There are many recipes for possets, both Tudor and Stuart. Like Sir Kenelm's tea, above, they could be taken as comfort food, easily digested and fortifying.

This receipt of Thomas Dawson's shows the transition between caudle and posset. It does not include cow's milk as many of the later possets do:

To make a Caudle to Comfort the Stomach, Good for an Old Man[51]
Take a pint of good muscadine, and as much of good stale ale, mingle
them together. Then take the yolks of twelve or thirteen eggs, new
laid. Beat well the eggs, first by themselves, [then] with the wine and
ale, and so boil it together. And put thereto a quartern [a quarter,
probably of a pound] of sugar, and a few whole mace, and so stir
it well, till it seethe [boil] a good while. When it is well sod, put
therein a few slices of bread if you will. And so let it soak a while,
and it will be right good and wholesome.

This would have turned into a curdled custard, tasting of wine
and ale but without the alcohol, which would have evaporated in
boiling. With luck it would have comforted the stomach of an old
woman, too. It sounds as if it would have been good for anyone
whose teeth had retired.

Special caudle cups were made for women to drink from after
childbirth, or for convalescents. They had two handles so that a
weak person could use both hands, but they had no foot, so that the
cup could not be set down until it was empty. Perhaps this would
have encouraged the invalid to drink up the contents completely.
Posset ale is mentioned quite frequently in both manuscripts and
printed books. Exactly what it was is not explained, but it seems
to be the result of mixing ordinary hot ale with eggs or milk, and
then straining it. '... take a quart of posset ale, the curde being well
drained from the same ...' says Markham in a drink for single tertian
fever [malaria].[52]

Mrs Corlyon too added herbs to posset ale to convert it into a
medicine:

A Possett Ale for the Coughe that commeth of an hott Rhewme[53]
Make a quart of cleare Possett Ale then take of Senneckle and
Foolefoote of eche an handfull, putt them into your Possett Ale with a
stick of Lycoresse, cleane scraped and brused. Boyle all these togeather
untill halfe a pinte be consumed, then putt it in a cleane pott, and
drinck thereof warmed in the morning fasting in the after noone and
at nighte when you goe to bedd but drincke it leasurely, and a good
quantity at a tyme and thus continue it as you shall fynde cause.

Possets later took a richer turn, with cream and wine. Several receipts say that the cream should be poured from a height, to make a froth. Mrs Miller has one such, made with sack, a wine similar to our sherry. It is not in the medical section of the notebook, but it would certainly be cheering. As the sack and ale were warmed but not boiled they would keep most of their alcohol.

To make a sack Possett[54]
Take 3 pints of Creame and sett it over the fire with on[e] Nutmegg sliced into itt stirring itt all the while then take 6 eggs and beate them very well and straine them and then take on[e] pinte of sacke and halfe a pint of Ale and a quarter of a pound of suger beat all these very well together in a bason over a Chaffing dish of Coales till they be all of a ffroth and then take the Creame from the fire and poure itt into them as high as ever you can and with as small a stream as may bee.

From here it is a small step to syllabub, though this was eaten cold. The Kidders give this delicious receipt.

To make a Syllabub[55]
Take three pints of sweet Creame and boyle it well with a sprigge of rosmary & a sl[i]ce of Lemone in it then lett it stand till it be but as warom as from the cow then take halfe a pint of white wine & the joice of two lemons sweetned with sugger then take the Creame & hould it as high as you can then pouer it in very sof[t]ly & when you have done lett it stand for three or [four] houers if it stands hafe a day it will be better

A well-fed body would be resistant to infection, a cheerful mind better able to cope with illness than a sad one. Restorative broths and nourishing drinks would really have helped a convalescent person to recover.

8

Women and
Children

It is difficult to talk about seventeenth-century women as if they were a homogeneous group. But it is possibly true to say that they were valued (by men) mostly for their ability to produce children and to serve the family, like Markham's ideal, by running a harmonious and comfortable household.

Inevitably the social position of a woman affected her work and outlook. For some rich ladies there was leisure, though even they were expected to carry out good works, and to run affairs at home when their husbands were away. For most women of the middling sort, life was probably hard, and though servants were comparatively cheap they were often young and needed training and supervision. Poor wives with children might have to help in field or workshop as well as look after the babies. But because a woman's primary function was childbearing, the womb was seen as her most important organ. Most feminine problems could be attributed to its various idiosyncrasies. 'It was the judgment of *Hippocrates*, that women's wombs are the cause of all their diseases; for let the womb be offended, all the faculties Animal, Vital and natural; all the parts, the Brain, Heart, Liver, Kidneys, Bladder, Entrails, and bones … partake with it.'[1]

So wrote Jane Sharp, who had had thirty years' experience when she published a book of good practice for midwives in 1671. She used contemporary sources as well as her own knowledge, but did not stray far from conventional theory. She had undoubted compassion for her patients, pointing out that they were more subject to disease than men, and 'great care should be had for the cure of that sex that is the weaker and most subject to infirmities ...' And what a list of infirmities! Just to start with there were '... white Feaver, or green Sickness, fits of the Mother, strangling of the Womb, Rage of the Matrix, extreme Melancholly, Falling-sickness, Head-ach ...'[2]

GREEN SICKNESS

Green sickness afflicted mostly young women. They were pale, and their skin had a greenish tinge. This gives the condition its other name of chlorosis. Further symptoms included lassitude or hysteria and strange food cravings which we should think indicated dietary deficiency. Contemporary opinions differed about the cause and cure. Jane Sharp attributes it to 'obstruction of the vessels of the womb, when the humours corrupt the whole mass of blood and over cool it, running back into the great veins.'[3] She had various complicated remedies, including marriage. Hannah Woolley however was decidedly unsympathetic:

> How to cure the Green-Sickness.[4]
> Laziness and love are the usual causes of these obstructions in young women; and that which increaseth and continueth this distemper, is their eating Oat-meal, chalk, nay some have not forebore Cinders, Lime, and I know not what trash. If you would prevent this slothful disease, be sure you let not those under your command to want imployment, that will hinder the growth of this distemper, and cure a worser Malady of a love-sick breast, for business will not give them time to think of such idle matters. But if this Green-sickness hath already got footing in the body, use this means to drive it away. Take a Quart of Claret-wine, one pound of Currans, and a handful of your Rosemary-tops, with half an ounce of Mace, seeth these to a pint, and let the Patient drink thereof three spoonfuls at a time, Morning and Evening, and eat some of the Currans after.

There is some iron in currants, and in red wine, so the concentrated claret might help, as it is now thought that green sickness was a form of anaemia.[5] If girls were not given enough iron-rich foods such as red meat and green vegetables, and if after menarche menstruation was heavy, it could well result in anaemia. It has also been suggested that the fashion for tight lacing may also have played a part.[6]

Lady Betty Egerton has an interesting remedy[7] which starts 'Steep an once [ounce] of hobnails in A quart of renish wine & let it steep 2 or 3 days before you take it then take 2 spoonsfuls of this wine every morning fasting ...' The hobnails gradually dissolved, because when the wine grew black the dosage was reduced to a single spoonful. Several other receipts dissolve steel filings in the same way. Whether the iron was in a form that the body could assimilate was another matter, but it was on the right track, an empirical treatment long before the idea of iron-deficiency had emerged.

MENSTRUAL PROBLEMS

Excessive menstrual bleeding could be a problem (especially perhaps in days before disposable sanitary protection had been invented). But, because there may be many causes, there was no certainty of cure. Gerarde suggests bistort root, a strong astringent, boiled in wine, to stop the bloody flux (dysentery) and 'it staieth also the ouer-much flowing of womens monethly sicknesses.'[8] On the other hand you might prefer a more folksy remedy:

> If a woman have too many flowres[9]
> Take the foot of an Hare, and put it in a new earthen pot, and burne it to powder, and let her drinke of that powder with warme ale, or with warme wine untill it be ceased.

This was an archaic belief. There was an almost identical receipt in a fifteenth century Leech book:

> An othir for to many floures for to cesse hem some Take an hare fote and brenne it to powdre and let hir drynke of that powder with stale ale first and last till she be hole.[10]

'Flowers' was a euphemism for menstruation. Hares are magical animals, associated both with luck and with witches. A hare's foot was usually carried as a charm, as Pepys did, but its occult properties evidently continued when reduced to powder, to dry the flowers by sympathy. At least in this form it would do no harm.

Markham had another, slightly more nourishing suggestion:

> To cesse women's flowers[11]
> Take the pouder of *Corrall* finely ground and eate it in a reare [rare, lightly cooked] egge, and it will stay the flux.

Or one could drink juice of plantain in red wine.

An opposite remedy might be needed, again for a variety of reasons. What we call amenorrhoea was taken seriously, because as Jane Sharp explains, menstruation was a way of purging the excess blood which in pregnancy would be used 'for the procreation and feeding of the Infant in the Womb.'[12] She had also said 'It is not onely blood is voided by the Terms, but a multitude of humours and excrements …'[13] These could give rise to many distressing complaints if retained in the body.

There was a connection with the moon. She says that young women had their courses 'when the Moon changeth, but women in years at the full of the Moon'. This is not especially noticed nowadays, so it is tempting to see a very old magical association of the moon with the first two of the three phases of female life: maiden, mother and crone. She mentions and partially refutes the ancient superstition about the menses, also mentioned by Pliny,[14] that:

> … some say this blood is venomous, and will poison plants it falls upon, discolour a fair looking glass by the breath of her that hath her courses, and comes but near to breath upon the Glass; that ivory will be obscured by it. It hath strong qualities indeed, when it is mixed with ill humours. But were the blood venomous it self, it could not remain a full month in the womans body, and not hurt her; nor yet the Infant, after conception, for then it flows not forth, but serves for the childs nutriment.[15]

She has a whole armoury of medicines to encourage restoration of the courses, including a mixture of syrups of mugwort, figwort, oximel (that is, honey and vinegar), and waters of motherwort, mugwort, pennyroyal and nip, all made into a julip to be drunk in three doses.[16] The most common reason for missed periods was of course pregnancy. Medicines which restored menstruation might do so by causing abortion, which was never openly advocated. Indeed, Jane Sharp warned against giving ointments, plasters and pessaries designed to promote menstruation to any woman with child 'for that will be Murder'. However, it would not take much imagination to apply these remedies illicitly to end an unwanted pregnancy. (See below on hindering conception too.)

The Mother

'The Mother', that is matrix or womb, could be a nuisance in many ways. It could become displaced, or cause 'Fits of the Mother', a mysterious complaint which seems to have afflicted many women. It apparently involved hysteria. All the collections have remedies for it. Hysteria was at one time thought to be caused by the womb moving upwards through the body due to the influence of malign humours. Originally attributed to Hippocrates, this idea was sometimes disputed during the seventeenth century. It was not altogether unreasonable. Prolapse of the uterus can certainly occur – 'Falling of the Mother' – so why not rising of the mother as well?

Mrs Corlyon has a pair of receipts to take care of these conditions:[17]

A Medecine for the fallinge of the Mother
First bathe the place very cleane with warme milke and presentlye after lay a plaister on the place made of blewe Beanes beaten to fyne flower, and then so much wine vineger as will make it spreade. Shifte it once euery 24. howers till it goe vpp.

A Medecine for the rysinge of the Mother
Take Chickweede and lay it as thick as your fingar and as longe and brode as a large hand, then laye on whole Mace on it, after more

Chickweede and more Mace and at last the Hearbe as at first. Then laye it to heate betweene two tyles till it be somewhat yeollowe and then in a thynn lynnen clothe laye it to the syde somethinge higher than the mother is and lett it lye 12. howers and it will very soone cause it to fall to the righte place. This is to be used eyther when the fitt is come, or that they feare the comminge of it.

Jane Sharp has a number of suggestions to persuade a fallen womb to return to its place, sensible ones which treat it like a rupture, and more questionable ones too, as if the womb were a semi-autonomous little animal: 'you may fright it in with a hot Iron presented near it as if you would burn it.'[18] A rising womb was more problematic: 'whether it can ascend and go upward is doubted by some; Physicians say it will if sweet things be held to the nose, if to the secrets it will fall downward; if stinking things be put to them it flyes from them ...' This was admittedly difficult to explain, as the womb was not able to 'smell scents no more than it can hear sounds or see objects ... but the womb partakes with these scents by reason of a thin vapour or spirit that comes from any strong smell ...' In the end it all depended on the status of the womb in relation to the good or ill humours it contained.[19]

Manipulation of the womb by scents appears in other receipts as well, as for instance in the following from the Barrett manuscript. Even if the womb itself was well anchored, vapours could still rise from it, to cause fits. The abdomen therefore needed to be constricted to restrain them. ('The vapours' continued to be the name given to tiresome episodes of female depression and hysteria right up to Victorian times):

For Fits of the Mother[20]
Take of assa foetida a scruple, of galbanum & opoponax of each 16 grains, of the powder of Castoreum of 10. grains, of rue seeds 8 grains, two drops of the oyl of Amber; & with the syrupe of May-wort, make small pills, whereof let the Patient take one, 3. or 4. times a day. Smelling to them is also usefull.
Give the Patient white wine to drink, being first powred through 5. or 6 balls of stone-horse dung, 2. or 3. times together.

Take a large silver Eele, & pull off the skin; w[hi]ch being cut open, applie the inward side thereof to the lower part of the bellie, fastning or sowing the same close behind on the woman's back. This will keep down the vapours, and not suffer them to rise above the ligature. The same growing drie, after 5 or 6 dayes wearing may be renewid. It is to be applied before the coming on of the fit & especially a day or two before the new & full moon.

This is interesting, not only because of the wandering vapours. The ingredients asafoetida, galbanum and opoponax are all strong-smelling resins derived from plants. Castoreum was also highly scented, a substance obtained from a particular kind of beaver. (These exotic ingredients were probably bought from the apothecary.) Smelling them would administer a kind of shock, just as smelling salts were used in a later period, and the taste of the pills would probably have been unpleasant too.

If this were not enough to keep the womb and vapours in their place, the unfortunate lady had to drink wine which had been filtered through horse dung. The receipt specifies the product of a stone-horse, that is a horse uncastrated, a full stallion. There seems to be an attempt to rebalance an excess of the female principle with an obvious symbol of maleness. It is just possible that the dung contained male hormone which might counteract overactive female hormones in pre-menstrual tension, though the species are incompatible.

The eel skin would dry and tighten round the woman's belly, to add to her discomfort until someone kindly replaced it after five or six days. Finally, there is again a clear connection between the woman's fits and the phases of the moon, the very ancient correspondence based on the cycle of about twenty-eight days common to both the moon and menstruation. It is also, perhaps, an echo of the astrology which was a feature of learned medieval medicine. The sub-text of this receipt is misogynistic.

Another antidote of maleness to counter female problems occurs in a different Barrett receipt, this time as an amulet:

For the mother & fainting[21]
Take a paire of Foxes Stones dry them & keep them in a little Bag &

hang them a bout the parties neck, soe th[a]t the bag be at the hole
of the Stomacke.
it is Dr Butlers receipt.

Hung at the level of the navel, near the womb, the testicles would
exert their power by propinquity. This remedy, and the following,
were both written by 'H. S.' who was, I believe, a woman:

For the Mother[22]
Take a quart of white wine, a quarter of a pinte of faire water, a
handful of maiden haire, fine loafe sugar ¼ of a pound. 10. damaske
pruins of endive succory, of each half a handfull, reasons of the sun
one handfull stoned. 3 dates sliced one nutmeg, one race of ginger,
one penny worth of sweet fennel Seeds, one good stick of english
lyquores all these must be boiled to a pint. take 3 spoonsfulls in the
morning & sleep, if you can after it & 3 spoonfulls at night when
you go to bed, and keep warme in the Chamber while you take it,
if one pint doe it not, take one pint more

Evidently this writer was far more sympathetic to women's problems. An extra snooze in bed sounds far better than a tight and
stinking eel-skin.

HELPING CONCEPTION

Fertility was important. At a time when infant and child mortality
was high, it was better to have too many children than too few, to
give the parents a sporting chance of raising at least some of them
to adulthood.

Infant mortality in the seventeenth century varied from about
150 to 300 per thousand births, depending partly on poverty, partly
on area, with the country literally a better place to live in.

John Graunt, an early pioneer of vital statistics, calculated that
out of every 100 live births, 36% would die before the age of six, with
a further twenty-four in the next ten years.[23] Thus less than half
the original number would survive to become adults. Admittedly

he was using the unreliable London Bills of Mortality, and it was known that cities were very unhealthy places. Even so, one can see why it was so desirable to conceive easily – if you could bear the heartache of losing children so often.

Markham recommends mugwort steeped in wine, or powdered mugwort and wine for 'Aptnes to conceiue'.[24] This might have been helpful in some cases, as it is an emmenagogue, normalising menstruation, as in the remedies cited above to restore the terms. It is also a general tonic. A panacea such as 'Dr Steevens Water' (see p. 51) was useful too. Among its many virtues 'It helpeth the conception of a Woman, if they be barren.'

The *Treasvrie of Hidden Secrets* has suggestions from early in the century as well (1637). I wonder what the *Polipi* were though. Octopus or squid might fit the description of 'many-feet', but these are hardly 'little'. Perhaps it meant sea-anemones, but this is a pure guess:

> *To make a barren woman beare children.*[25]
> Take of these little sea-fishes, called in Latine *Polipi*, or *Polipodes*, and rost them upon the Embers without Oyle, and let the woman eat of them, and it shall profit and helpe her very much, having in the meane time the company of a man.

Maybe both partners needed feeding up a bit, to give them vigour:

> To strengthen the seed.[26]
> Take Succory, Endive, Plantin, Violet flowers and the leaves, Clary, Sorrell, of each half an handfull, with a peece of Mutton, make a good broth, and to eate it evening and morning is speciall good.

HINDERING CONCEPTION

Family planning is not a modern idea. Some people have always preferred not to have children at all. Even Jane Sharp concedes that 'Virginity and single life in some cases, is preferred before Matrimony, because it is a singular blessing and gift of *God*,'[27] but the only acceptable means to ensure celibacy was prayer and fasting. She says that '*Nuns*, and such as cannot marry, may use things, [t] hat by a hidden quality diminish seed, but they cause barrenness: let them eat no eggs, nor much nourishing meats, and sleep little.'[28]

Nevertheless, Gerarde mentions an intriguing herb, 'Barren woort' which 'some authors affirme, being drunke is an enimie to conception.'[29] Maybe his sources were mistaken though, or he meant something else than the plant which a modern herbal identifies as barrenwort, *Epimedium saggitarium*, or horny goat weed, an aphrodisiac![30]

He mentions another plant too, *Agnus castus* or the Chaste Tree[31] This was:

> ... a singular medicine and remedie for such as would willingly liue chaste, for it withstandeth all vncleannes, or desire to the flesh, consuming and drying vp the seede of generation, in what sort soever it be taken ... [in powder or decoction] or whether the leaues be caried about the body ...

Most of this is confirmed by the same modern herbal. *Agnus castus* does have a hormonal effect which reduces libido,[32] — though the power of its leaves as an amulet is perhaps exaggerated.

PREGNANCY

Pregnancy was hazardous:

> As for women with child they are subject to miscarry, to hard labour, to disorderly [abnormal] births of their children, sometimes the child is dead in the womb; sometimes alive, but must be taken forth by cutting or the woman cannot be delivered; sometimes she is troubled with false conceptions, with ill formations of the child, with superfetations, another child begot before she is delivered of her first; with monsters or Moles [severely malformed foetuses] and many more such like infirmities.[33]

The advice in the household notebooks is profuse, from normal management of pregnancy and delivery to distinctly pathological events.

Woolley's advice 'To preserve the Infant, and prevent Abortion' is to:

> take Coriander-seed prepared two drams, of the roots of Bistort, the shaving of Ivory, & red Coral, of each a dram, of white Amber and Crystal, of each a Scruple, Alkermes [a sweet red cordial] half a Scruple, Sugar dissolv'd in four Ounces of Rose-water; make tables [tablets] each of them weighing a dram[34]

Two of these were to be taken every other day. The precious ingredients, ivory, coral, amber and crystal have a distinctly magical aura. This was precious medicine for a precious child. Similar ingredients went into 'An Excellent Cordiall Powder' in Barrett, used to prevent flux.[35] (See also Chapter 12.)

There is a delicious receipt in *The Queen's Closet* 'To preserve a woman with Childe from miscarrying and Abortion'.[36] It starts:

> Take a Fillet of Beef half roasted hot from the fire, then take half a pinte of Muscadine [wine], Sugar, Cinnamon, Ginger, Cloves, Mace, Graines of Paradise and Nutmegs, of each half a dram, and make thereof a Sawce, then divide the Beef into two pieces and wet them in the sawce ...

You might think that the woman and her husband, or even the woman and her midwife, would then sit down to a good nourishing meal of rare fillet steak. But no:

> ... and binde the one peece to the bottome of the womans belly, and the other to the Reins of the Back [kidney area], as hot as may be suffered, and keep them on twenty four hours at the least, and longer if need be thereof.

CHILDBIRTH

If pregnancy in general was perceived as hazardous, childbirth was even worse.

> And as for women in child-bed, sometimes the *Secundine* or after-birth will not follow, their purgations [lochia] are too few or too many, they are in great pains in their belly, their privities are rended by hard delivery as far as their Fundament, also they are inflamed many times and ulcerated and cannot go to stool [open their bowels] but their fundament will fall forth. They have swoonding and epileptick fits, watching [sleeplessness] and dotings, their whole body swels, especially their belly, legs and feet: they are subject to hot sharp Feavers and acute diseases, to vomiting and costiveness, to fluxes, to incontinence of Urine, that they cannoth hold their water.[37]

Though high by today's standards, the number of women who actually died in labour was not, according to Graunt, excessively high. He remarks:

> In regular times, when accounts were well kept, we find, that not above three in 200 died in childbed, and that the number of abortives [stillborn] was about treble to that of the women dying in childbed: from whence we may probably collect [understand] that not one woman of an hundred (I may say of two hundred) dies in her labour; forasmuch as there be other causes of a woman's dying within the month, than the hardness of her labour.[38]

The 'other causes' would have included puerperal fever, not separately mentioned in the Bills, but probably contributing to the high numbers of those dead from fevers in general. To illustrate these trends, in 1678 there were 12,601 christenings, 272 women who died in childbed, 710 cases of abortion and stillbirth, and 301 'chrisomes and infants' who died in the first month of life. The figure for ague and fever lumped together was 2,376 but this did not include specific fevers such as smallpox and spotted fever.

There were several ways of assisting labour. For instance Grace Acton has an early folk-remedy:

> To ease a woman big wythe childe[39]
> Straddle a pot of boiling seewater to whych has been added vitriol and soot from a fire repeat til the childe be delivered.

The warm steam might help to relax the woman, though if vitriol was the same then as now I wouldn't try it myself.

Markham has an interesting one:

> For ease in child bearing.[40]
> If a woman haue a strong and hard labour: take iiij spoonefull of another womans milke, and giue it the woman to drinke in her labour, and shee shall be deliuered presently [at once].

There might be a hormonal reason for this effect, but it could work by suggestion too. The donor of the milk had done it and come through, so why not the woman in travail?

Jane Sharp's herbal helps were syrups of featherfew [feverfew] and mugwort, or powdered cinnamon in wine or distilled water of various birth-herbs, including pennyroyal, or powders also including pennyroyal and round birthwort. Magical help was at hand if one could get hold of an eagle-stone (see p. 190).[41] Gerarde suggested rue – useful of course against poison – but also to help women, as it 'bringeth down the sicknes [menstruation], expelleth the dead childe and afterbirth, being inwardly taken, or the decoction drunke …'[42] It is an emmenogogue, and in large doses can cause abortion, so it was probably effective to make the womb contract.

After being delivered, the mother might have after-pains, which could be helped by plenty of beer boiled with camomile-flowers. If she was fainting or swooning, a handful of mugwort, motherwort and mint could be stewed in a pint of malmsey, and taken in doses of two or three spoonfuls.[43] Motherwort contains a heart stimulant, so this makes sense.

After labour, the woman would need to sleep, but might need help. Here is F. Head, in the Barrett manuscript:[44]

To Ease pain, & cause sleep, p[re]scribed to my wife, when she lay in.
Cowslip flowers an handfull, of anise-seeds & juniper berries a little bruised & licourish of each 20. graynes (or 30.) boyle these in Milke (in 6.ounces of milke) with small beere make it a posset, strayne it, take 3 ounces & an half of it, and colour it a little with a grayne or two of dried Saffron, adding thereunto half an ounce or 5. drachmes of the syrrup of white poppie./. by S[i]r G. Ent

Cowslip flowers contain a sedative, and poppy is soporific, so Sir George Ent was on the right lines here. He was an eminent practitioner, a founder-member of The Royal Society. He was evidently respected by the Head family, as several receipts are ascribed to him. This is also an example of how the physician influenced household remedies at times. (Occasionally there are prescriptions which could only be made up by an apothecary, but it was clearly useful to have them on record.)

NURSING, SORE BREASTS

There are numerous receipts to increase milk in nursing mothers and wet nurses. Markham[45] suggests colewort − a sort of cabbage − boiled in posset ale, the ale to be drunk at every meal. Colewort served with meat 'will wonderfully increase her milke also'. Perhaps we would say that the woman's diet needed improvement. Woolley suggests:

> An infallible receipt to increase milk in Womens breasts.[46]
> Take Chickens and make broth of them, then add thereunto Fennel and Parsnip-roots, then take the newest-made Butter you can procure, and butter the roots therewith; having so done let her eat heartily, and her expectations therein will be speedily satisfied.

One of the consequences of lactating might be sore breasts, and many remedies are given. This is one of the simplest, from Barrett:

The Ale-Salve, for a sore breast[47]
Boyle a Gallon of the newest thickest Ale, till it comes to a
Consistencie that it will spread upon the rough side of Leather. Cut
an Hole for the Nipple, & applie it to the breast.

If it was necessary to stop the flow of milk, Mrs Corlyon suggests
a kind of lead brassière: 'Make thinn Boales [bowls] of Leade fitt to
couer the Brest … and when you do lay it to the Breste warme it a
litle and so … make it fast that it remoue not and lett it lye as you
feele occasion …'[48]

THE NEWBORN CHILD

As soon as the child is born, according to Jane Sharp, the navel string
(umbilical cord), should be bound with a ligature to prevent blood
and the vital spirits being lost, and then cut. If the child was weak,
the cord could be pressed gently first to give the baby the maximum
benefit of the blood it contained. Or six or seven drops of blood
from the cord could be given by mouth.[49]

Convulsions in the newborn infant were feared, with reason,
and blood from the umbilical cord was thought to be protective.
Perhaps the blood which had sustained the child in the womb would
continue to exert power:

To Keep a Child from convulsion or other Fitts.[50]
The first thing that you ever give it, take one drop of that bloud that
comes from the nauell [navel] strings, & mingle with it in the spoon
a little sack. This is by Experience proued verie good.

An alternative in the same Barrett manuscript, but in a different, less
educated hand, is a straightforward herbal medicine, which would
have had a laxative effect:

To give a Child when it is new born to prevent fits.[51]
Take two drams of Oyle of sweet almons, (new drawn) a dram &
half of surrup of Succory with Rubbub, & 3 or 4 drams of Cinamon

Water & mix these & give the Child half, & two or three howers
after give the rest to the Child, before any other food.

Parents then, as now, did not appreciate broken nights. Here is an
early form of gripe water, with soporific poppy:

For a Griping in a child, & to cause sleep.[52]
Take one spoonfull of Garden Poppie syrrup, add 3. spoonfulls of
Spare-Mint [spearmint] water stilled in a cold still, mingle them
well, & sweeten it well with Sugar. Give it a spoonfull ever[y] night,
the last thing he eats.

CHILDISH DISEASES

Graunt's calculations led him to say that over 20 years, out of a
total mortality of 229,250, there were 71,124 deaths from 'Thrush,
convulsion, rickets, teeth and worms, and as abortives, chrysomes,
infants, livergrown and overlaid; that is to say that about 1/3 of
the whole died of those diseases, which we guess did all light upon
children under four or five years old.'

Thrush is a fungal infection, which might have given babies
and young children problems when they tried to swallow. Worm-
remedies have been described on p. 114.

Teething does not cause death, but because babies and toddlers
spend a lot of time with erupting teeth, it was no doubt easy to
attribute what we call an acute infection to this cause. Jane Sharp
remarks that 'Children are subject to all sorts of Feavers, but chiefly
to Feavers from corrupt milk, and Feavers with breeding of teeth.'
(She goes on to mention measles and smallpox 'all children almost
will have them first or last.'[53]) Just as an example, in 1678 the Bill of
Mortality gave the number of those dying of 'Teeth' as 1110, although
some of them *might* have been adults with severe dental problems.

Mrs Corlyon has a receipt which would have caused distraction
for the child, even if it didn't do much to encourage the teeth to
come through. Toadflax can be used as a poultice,[54] perhaps used
here to cool the skin:

For a soore mouthe happening to Children when they breede Teethe[55]
Take a pretty quantitye of Toadeflaxe otherwise called Staggerworte: Bruse the greene thereof very well in your hand, and lay a good quantitye of the same vnder the chynn and Iawes [jaws] of the Childe fasten it w[i]th a clothe and chaunge it once in 12. or 24. howers as you fynde occasion.

Rickets is a condition in which the bones do not develop properly, leading to late walking, bow legs, swollen joints, sometimes a large head and twisted spine. It persisted as a childhood disease up to the early twentieth century, when it was shown to be due to a deficiency of vitamin D. Adequate sunlight on the skin makes the body produce its own vitamin D, and it is present in whole cow's milk, butter, cheese and especially cod-liver oil, not of course available as such in the seventeenth century. Babies who were weaned late, and toddlers who were fed mainly on starchy pap would be vulnerable, especially as there was no tradition of letting children run about in the sunshine with bare arms and legs. Charles I was a rachitic child, and aristocratic infants were probably worse off than poor children playing in the fields as their mothers worked. There was no humoral explanation for the condition, as it did not appear in Galen.

The Queen's Closet has three receipts, Hannah Woolley one. Three out of the four are for various unguents and rubs – you could anoint your child with the liquid from squashed garden snails, or butter mixed with pounded sanicle and red mints[56] or thickened juice of marjoram and sage, made into an ointment with ox-marrow.[57] The fourth receipt, from *The Queen's Closet*, would have far more chance of living up to the claim that it had been found effective:

To cure the Rickets in Children. Approved.[58]
Take a quart of new Milk, put into it one handful of Sanicle, boyl it half away, and give it the patient child to drink in the morning for a breakfast, and let it not eat any thing for an hour or two after it and at night take a quart of Milk and one handful of red Mints, boyl it half away as before and let the child eat it last at night. This

continue for a month, or longer, as occasion is. The quantity of milk so made, will serve for twice.

The seventeenth-century woman, whatever her status, had to endure very many 'griefs' in all senses, from puberty to the menopause. Marriage and childbirth were what she had been brought up to expect and welcome. She deserved the several weeks' holiday of her lying-in after she had given birth, before the whole process was repeated. She could hardly hope that all her children would live, and she herself could think herself lucky if she survived into real old age.

9
Old Age

THE ANCIENT BODY

How old is old? The concept changes from century to century. With improved living standards and all the medical discoveries of the last 400 years, most of us in the privileged developed world can now hope to live into our eighties.

With lives no longer halted abruptly by pneumonia, smallpox, plague, puerperal fever and so on, degenerative diseases now have more chance to manifest themselves in older bodies. But there were, of course, some survivors to old age in the past, and they suffered from such conditions as aches and swellings of joints, shrunken sinews, dropsy (most likely caused by heart disease), kidney and bladder problems, including the stones which could occur at any age, difficulty in passing urine, gout, palsy, paralysis and loss of speech, probably caused by strokes. There was not much to be done, really, for this suffering, except palliative care, and the restorative cordials and broths, described in Chapters 3 and 7, to cheer and nourish.

ACHES AND PAINS, SCIATICA

There was a huge range of ointments, oils, salves, searcloths and poultices which could be tried for aches and swellings. Mrs Corlyon can be relied upon to come bustling up with treatments for all occasions. Many ointments were made by letting mashed herbs stand in some kind of fat, then boiled and strained. Here is one example, with several uses:

An Oyntement of St Johns woorte good for all Aches, and is good eyther of it selfe or to be putt in Salues for watering Soores. It is also good for any Pricke or greene Wounde[1]
Take of St Johns woorte a weeke before Midsommer or a weeke after stripe it from the Stalkes, choppe it smale, stampe it with freshe Hogges grease temper it like doughe and putt it into an earthen pott and so lett it stand and rott the space of a fortenighte or 3. weekes Then boile it vppon a soft fyer the space of an hower and after straine it and so putt it vpp into a Vessell and keepe it for your vse.

She has a general purpose ointment for 'all kinde of Aches and Bruses',[2] made from sage, rue, wormwood and bay leaves, sheep's fat, and olive oil. It was left to mature for eight days, then boiled and strained like the St John's wort. The grease and oil would have absorbed some of the fat-soluble components of the herbs, so the method made sense.

Others were far less pleasant. The Kidders, at the end of the century, have a barbaric one. (Cat-lovers can skip this receipt, reminiscent of a witch's pharmacopoeia):

An excellent oyle for an ache[3]
Take an ould fatt bore Catt and Case [skin] him then take a handfull of Rosemary a handfull of herbe of grace then gather snayles enough to fill the belly of the catt and stampe the herbes and snayles altogather powering [pouring] aquavitty on as you stampe them and then fill the Catts bellye and rost him without basteing and resarue the oyle or drippings and anoynet the grieued place therewith probatum Est

I think there is a definite waste of aquavitae here.

Mrs Corlyon's remedy for 'Syatica in the hipp Bone',[4] that sounds very much like modern arthritis, was to rub it well with black soap, in front of the fire, 'bothe euening and morninge and in a fewe dressinges it will procure ease.' *The Queen's Closet* takes up the idea, but makes a poultice of black soap, oatmeal and mutton fat for an ache or swelling.[5]

Both Mrs Corlyon and Gerarde[6] use horse-radish to apply to painful joints. Horse-radish when crushed or scraped produces a pungent substance, like mustard, that will redden or even blister the skin.

The sensation of heat, and increased blood-flow, may have helped. Rubefacient creams are still prescribed for painful joints.

Shrunken or Broken Sinews

What was meant by this is puzzling, as we have no modern equivalent, unless it is the deformity caused by advanced arthritis. The remedy, sadly, sometimes involved nestling swallows made into an ointment with lavender cotton, strawberry runners and other herbs, boiled in May butter.[7] There may have been magical thinking here. The young swallows might cause renewal. So too might earthworms, with their partial ability to regenerate when damaged. First catch your worms ... but don't expect them to co-operate:

> For Sinews that be Broken in Two[8]
> Take worms while they be nice, and look that they depart not. Stamp them, and lay it to the sore, and it will knit the sinew that be broken in two.

Gerarde however has an internal remedy, tansy seeds pounded and mixed with olive oil, against 'the paine and shrinking of the sinews'. Fresh young tansy leaves were the main ingredient of a dish of the same name, a kind of herb omelet, made in the spring and eaten to purge the stomach. 'For if any bad humors cleave thereunto, it doth perfectly concoct them ['cook' or digest them] and scowre them downwards.' If gout was the problem, tansy root preserved with honey or sugar was an especially good thing.[9]

Gout

Gout, we now know, is caused by a metabolic disorder, in which salts of uric acid build up in the joints, especially in the big toe joints. It is painful, with swelling and inflammation. Because of the sensation of heat, it seemed likely to the Galenist that a hot humour was involved, though there was also another manifestation of gout which came of a cold humour. Purgation was the remedy in any case for Hannah Woolley (and perhaps for Gerarde, as above):

> The Gout whether hot or cold, or of whatever temperature, ariseth from one and the same cause, though the effects seem different. As for example, Fat-men have it with much inflammation, redness and great pain, in leaner Persons it is discovered with less inflammation, though not with lesser pain; it afflicteth Cholerick and Melancholick men with nodes and tumors The cause of this distemper cometh from an evil quality engendred in the Stomack, Blood and Liver, the cure therof must be then the removal of this ill quality from the Stomack, and the purgation of Blood and Liver ... [10]

There was a poultice alternative to treatment by internal medicine or ointment. Mrs Corlyon's remedy had the benefit of being made from cheap ingredients readily available in the country:

> A Medecine for the Goute that commeth of an hott Humer. It will ease the paine and coole the heate[11]
> Take of Cowe dounge when it is new made and putt thereto so much of new milke from the Cowe, as will make it somewhat thynn Stirr them well togeather and boyle it vppon a softe fyer vntill it be thicke, then spredd it vppon a clothe and lay it to the place greeued, as warme as the Patient can endure it. Shifte it once in 24. howers, and in short tyme it will ease. Vse this as you do fynde occasion.

Was there was some special virtue in animal dung, besides availability? I shall return to this question later, in Chapter 12. In this case it was possibly useful to hold the comforting heat, though not, one would have thought, for twenty-four hours at a time. The Kidders are still using the same kind of thing later in the century, with this receipt already mentioned in Chapter 1:

> A most Excelent Bath for the Goute or lameness by salte humers[12]
> Take sage worm[wo]od and fennell prim Rose roots burdock Roots mallowes costmary Burdock juce when the leaves are in the prime and boyle the herbes and Roots in the Burdock juce which you

may keep all the year with sallet oyle there and a large quantity of urin[e] and good large quantity of ston[e] horse Dung and give all a good boyle togeather and have a tubb like a butter Firkin soe high that the bath may reach your knees & sitt with your leggs only in it for an hour in the day for 10 days it will sartainly Qure the goute though in the handes or armes as well as legges onely by sitting in it

Perhaps it would have been preferable to go back to another of Mrs Corlyon's receipts:

A Medecine good for the Gowte and to drawe out all euell Humors from any parte of the Bodye. Also very good to amende the Sighte, ease any paine in the Heade, breake any Impostume, and to take away defectes in hearinge.[13]

Take two pounde of Pitche, as much of Rozen as much of Frankensence eche fynelye beaten and searzed seuarallye, one pounde of Sheepes tallowe one ownze of Saffron two ownzes of Cloues, as much of Mace, halfe a pounde of Commyn and 3. ownzes of Lapdanum [a gum] beaten and searzed. All these muste be sodden the space of an hower The Pitche must be putt in first alone, and after the rest, and when it is sodden, make it in longe rolles and keepe it Then to use it take fyne tawed Sheepes leather and thereof cutt Sooles to couer the Sooles of your feete, and spreade of the foresaid Plaister vppon them and weare them next your feete within your Sockes the space of a monethe or vntill they fall of[f] and use them so longe as you fynde occasion or ar thereunto disposed.

Medicinal insoles, with possibly the absorption of some component of the pitch, seems to be an inspiration which owes a lot to counter-magic. If there is some kind of grief in the head, a foot treatment might draw the evil humour downwards. If the gout was in the foot, the application might directly affect the pain. As it is phrased, it sounds as if you might wear your socks until they fall off of their own accord. It is tempting to wonder if this might be a distant foreshadowing of New Age reflexology. In any case the idea of treating one part of the body by putting a poultice on another part is like the wrist-plaster described on p. 75.

All these aches and pains and ills of joints and sinews seem to have been common. The housewife would do well to have a general purpose ointment in her store cupboard. Forethought was important. Each season had its tasks, and in summer one made remedies like the following, taking advantage of flowers as they came into bloom. With luck the ointment would last for several years:

An Oyntement called Oyle of Exeter[14]
Take in the moneth of Maye a pounde of the flowers of Coweslypps and steepe them in Oyle Oliue, as much in quantity as they may easely be laid in. Then take Calamynte Hearbe Iohn, Sage Turmentill Sothernewoode woormewood Pennyroyall Lauender Pellitory of Spaine Peritorye [sic, repeat?] Rosemary Camomele Heryffe Leaues of Lawrye flowers of Lillies of eyther an handfull gathered in the monethe of Iune Grynde them in a morter as smale as it were for sawse, then take the flowers abouesaid and wringe them out of the Oyle with cleane handes, put them in a morter with the other hearbes and grinde them togeather, that doen putt them into so much white wine as they may easelye be steeped in and lett it lye there 24 howers in a vessell cloose stopped. Then take the hearbes with the wine and the Oyle of Oliue that the flowers were steeped in and lett them boile on a softe fyer togeather till the wine and the water of the hearbes be wasted awaye (w[hi]ch you may thus knowe, take a spoonefull of the lyquor that is in the Pannes bottome and if you can discerne no water in the Spoone it is boyled enoughe) Then take it of the fyer and caste it im[m]ediatelye into a bagg of stronge newe canuas and straine it forceablye betweene two staues. Putt it vpp in a vessell of Tynn or Glasse for no other kinde of vessell will containe it so well, and keepe it for your vse. This Oyle or Oyntement maybe applied and wilbe auaileable to such places of Man or Woeman as ar brused with Goutes or Palsyes. In Sommer annoynte in the warme Sonn and in Winter by the fyer. And after the annointinge laye on the place blacke woole that neuer was washed made hott againste the fyer. This Oyntement is good against all manner of Malladyes that be in the Synewes by occasion of any colde and is remeadiable for all bruses of Bones and Ioyntes. It must be made vpp in the moneth of Iune for all the yeare after and with good keepinge it will continue good 3. yeares.

STONE AND GRAVEL

Stones in kidney or bladder seem to have been especially trouble-some in the seventeenth century, possibly because of recurrent infections, faulty diet or insufficient liquid intake resulting in high concentrations of minerals in the urine. Stones form when crys-tals precipitate out of a strong solution. A clump of dead cells or bacteria, even a small blood clot, can form a nucleus, and thus a small stone gradually gets bigger as more and more mineral salts are deposited. Although stones can form in young people as well as old, they are more likely to appear in the elderly, and have a connection with gout. Stones in kidneys cause pain, especially if they obstruct the ureter or travel through it to the bladder. Bladder stones are similarly distressing and dangerous.

Pepys was famously 'cut for the stone' as a young man, and lived to celebrate every year the anniversary of his deliverance from the debilitating pain. At a cost of twenty-five shillings, a lot of money, he had a case made for his stone,[15] and displayed it to interested friends. He was lucky as well as brave. There were specialist sur-geons for the operation, but many people died of it all the same.

Gravel was a collection of small stones which could sometimes pass naturally out of the body. One of the household treatments for stone or gravel was based on flushing them out. Others attempted to break or dissolve them. As usual Mrs Corlyon has a large number of helpful suggestions. Among these are several distilled waters, a syrup or conserve of sea-holly, wild rose hips and winter cherries,[16] a preventative broth 'to keepe the Backe from slymye causes and from the breeding of the Stone'[17] and a 'Quintasye for the Stone'.[18] A quintessence was, as we might say, the very best medicine. It was a mixture of a pint each of nine different waters already distilled from herbs and flowers and another nine pints of Muscatel wine. This was distilled again until two quarts had been drawn off, to be kept separately from what was left. These first two quarts were the quintessence:

> ... And when you will use these waters Lett the Patient troubled
> with the Stone take halfe a pinte of the Quintessence and a whole

pinte of the other water, and lett hym drinck of eyther the said halfe
pinte or the whole pinte, or as much thereof as he is able to drinck,
and lett hym walke after it holdinge his water as much as he can, and
when he can holde it no longer to make it with as greate force as he
can. you must take but halfe the quantity in the eueninge and then
he shall not neede to walke so longe after it before he takes his reste.

Some receipts are based on fruit stones themselves. For example:

for the stone[19]
take powder of olive stone or powder of cheery stons and drinke it
in Ale and it is very good.

The Barrett manuscript has a slightly different slant, with the gum
of plum trees dissolved in hot milk, and 'drink it as hot as you can
endure it, and this wil draw away the Stone in the Blader.'[20]

However, it is Edward Kidder, who wrote the notebook with his
wife, who gives a cure from personal experience. (His enthusiasm
is not matched by his punctuation, but like Pepys he is interested in
what he produced.)

A receet for an excelent cure for the gravill[21]
Take the hard rowes of three red herrings & the shells of fife new
laid egs drie them slowly in an ouen or before a fier fitt to be made
powder of then pound them in a morter and sift them throw a fine
siue then grate a larg nutmeg into it then take one ounc of it then
take one ounc of the sorope of allthea [marsh mallow] and one ounc
of the sorope of sweet allmondes & as much as will lie on a shilling
of the pouder & mix with the 2 former liquids into half a pint of
whit wine warom & drink it of[f] doe this four ouer three or fore
times & it is infallable to cure the grauell when you make wather
lett it be in a clean pot and lett it setle & you will find the grauill in
the bott [sic, bottom] of the pott this is Capt[ain] Kidder his Recept

Retention of urine is always serious, no matter what the cause,
which might be stone, tumour, enlarged prostate and so on. Captain
Kidder suggests you take '7 bees from the hive drye them and beate

them to powder and give the partye to drinke in a pint of ordinarye stale beere.'[22] Seven is a magic number, and there are many superstitions associated with bees, but why powdered bees should improve this complaint is puzzling.

DROPSY

Dropsy is the accumulation of fluid in the body. One common cause is a heart that can no longer cope with its burden, and begins to fail. The seventeenth-century household books, even later ones, take no notice of William Harvey's work on the circulation of the blood, and the importance of the heart. Dropsy is seen as a separate disease or condition. There was a surgical procedure where fluid was drawn off in some cases,[23] but the housewife used herbal drinks, baths and ointment. Mrs Corlyon has two medicines, one a strong infusion of guaiacum wood made into ale, another with elecampane, wormwood, rue, lovage, aniseed, liquorice, honey, and a small quantity of 'Colloquintida', which might have been colocynth, a poisonous pulp with drastic water-removing properties.[24] There were also baths for the legs[25] and an ointment made of herbs and May butter.

Both Hannah Woolley and the Kidders have receipts using the ashes of green broom. Hannah boils the ashes in wine, which is then strained and taken three times a day, 'which has cured many a Person when they were left and forsaken by Physicians'.[26] The Kidders have a cold infusion of the ashes in Rhenish wine, with wormwood, centaury and gentian.[27] It is possible that burning concentrated some minerals in the plant.

It was to be about another hundred years before a country herbal tea for treating swollen legs was investigated by William Withering. He published his findings in 1785, showing that the foxglove (which contained digitalis) stimulated the heart and reduced the dropsy.[28] Gerarde had missed this. He said that foxgloves:

> in that they are bitter, are hot and dry, with a certaine kinde of clensing qualitie joyned therewith; yet are they of no use, neither have they any place amongst medicines, according to the Antients.[29]

PALSY, PARALYSIS, LOSS OF SPEECH

It isn't entirely clear what was meant by 'palsy' in the receipts. The term seems to cover both tremor and paralysis, and malaise felt in the head. We should attribute paralysis to brain disease or injury, but it was not until the later part of the century, with the work of Dr Thomas Willis, that neurology began to be studied scientifically. Nevertheless, in the receipts the palsy is often connected with the head. In the early part of the century Mrs Corlyon has, as might be expected, medicines, drinks, waters and ointment. The following is a general-purpose remedy for unease in the head. The 'colde' mentioned is most probably a cold humour, not our cold-in-the-head with stuffy nose and sneezes:

> The makinge of a water for the Palsye. It is good also to quicken Memorye and to cheare the Sighte[30]
> Take of Prymerose flowers, with the younge leaues and buddes of the flowers and budds of Coweslipps, of Rosemary flowers and buddes and of the flowers and budds of Hartesease otherwise called Wall Gyllyflowers Of eche of these the like quantitye, then take as much of Balme as of all the other, mingle all these togeather and when they are somewhat dryed, distyll them and vse the water as you woulde doe other distilled waters, then keep it for your vse And take thereof when you doe feele eyther lightnesse in your heade or coldnesse or any other paine w[hi]ch commeth of colde in your heade And as you do take it holde some in your mouthe that the Sente may assende into your heade and you shall fynde ease therebye.

More problematic to us is the connection of foxes with palsy:

> An approued Medecine for the Palsye[31]
> Take a Foxe and vncase [skin] hym then mynse his fleshe as smale and as fyne as is possible, then take a fatt Goose and scalde her very cleane and plucke out her guttes and fyll her Bellye w[i]th the same mynsed Foxe and sowe vpp the hoole againe that none come out. Putt her vppon a spitt and rost her well and keepe the drippinge

thereof cloose in a neyled [annealed, perhaps glazed] pott and an-
noyte the place therewith where the greefe is and chafe it by the fyer.

Gervase Markham remarks 'For the *Apoplexie* or palsy the strong
scent or smell of a Fox is exceeding soueraigne,' though you might
also drink distilled lavender water and rub the head twice a day with
a rough cloth, 'whereby the humors may be dissolued and disperst
into the outward parts of the body ...'[32] The fox/goose ointment
presumably worked in the same way, by dispersing the humour
causing the grief.

Dr Stevens Water (p. 51) was another alternative according to
The Queen's Closet, as it 'helpeth the shaking of the palsie'.[33] This is a
clue that this palsy might be something like our Parkinson's Disease.

A little later Mrs Miller was making 'The Palsey water, alsoe for
Apoplexies or distempers or ffumes in the head',[34] a very complicated remedy with lavender flowers soaked in wine or aquavitae,
distilled after six weeks. To this was added flowers of sage, rosemary, bittony, borage, bugloss, lilies, and cowslips and left to 'digest'
in a warm place for another six weeks. Then she added balm, motherwort and spike (lavender) flowers, with bay leaves cut small, leaves
and blossom of orange trees. This was distilled once more. So it goes
on with added ingredients and repeated distillation – dried citrus
peels, peony seeds, jujubes, aloe wood, spices – until the 'water' was
finally strained, but still had prepared pearl, two drams of ambergris,
and the same quantity of 'dead mens skulls in fine powder', saffron
and saunders, both yellow and red, to be put into a bag and soaked
in it for a further three weeks in a close-stopped vessel:

> ... When you finde any indisposition or ffear of any fitt take of this
> water a Little spoonfull with white bread Crums or alone itt helps
> all Palseys in what kinde soever though on[e] bee quite given over
> for dead and itt Restores the Limbs Bathed with itt, and ye speech
> though Lost. for prevention take of this water Euery other Chang[e]
> of the moon. Probatum Est The Lady ffaulconbridge

A great deal of time had gone into obtaining the herbs at the proper
seasons, preparing all this and keeping an eye on the liquid while it

was standing about in a warm place. It might have fermented and blown off the stopper. Then there was the expense of the precious ingredients. In 1676 ambergris cost twenty shillings a dram,[35] that is one-eighth of an ounce, so this had forty shillings' worth. The dead men's skulls in powder connect this recipe to others for diseases of the head, such as epilepsy, which I shall be looking at later (p. 185). It is linked to the idea that the moon was influential too, in diseases of the brain or head. This was a very precious medicine, for desperate conditions. You would make it up in advance, ready to restore the senior members of your family after doctors had given up, or to prevent them getting into this state in the first place.

Poorer people stricken with paralysis, perhaps after a stroke, could try a more economical remedy, like this from the Barrett manuscript. It seeks to make matters better by treating the afflicted limb, not the head or brain:

An Oyntment for one that has lost the use of their limbs[36]
Of stale strong beere a quart, of red sadg a handfull boile this together till it coms to a pint, then straine it hard out, & put it into a new pipkin, & add to it 4 ounces of butter without salt & let it boile together a little while, when you take it off, add to it half a quarter of a pint of brandy, then anoint the limbs 3 mornings.
This receit cured a man t[ha]t could neither stand nor goe

Loss of speech was blamed partly on a dysfunction of the tongue, but a connection was also made with palsy, even with mental trauma. Mrs Corlyon of course has a remedy ...

A Medecine for those that haue lost theire Speeche eyther by Sicknesse feare or otherwise[37]
Take a Prynerose roote [sic], Scrape it cleane, then take a slyce of the inner part of it, of a good thicknes and putt it vnder the Patientes tounge. Then annoynte the Noddell of his heade, the Nape of his neck and about his eares and iawes with the Oyntement for the Palsye (w[hi]ch you shall fynde written in this Booke) chafe it well and lapp a clothe about it beynge but warmed at the fyer and so lapp it vpp close with sufficient clothes to keepe it warme. Dresse hym

thus once in twelve howers, and continue as you shall see occasion: to[o] much heate of the fyer is hurtefull, to those that have the Palsye but competent warmeth is good.

The Queen's Closet has a simpler suggestion 'For one that hath no Speech in sickness' juice of sage or pimpernel put in the mouth, 'and by the grace of God it shall make him speak.' The next receipt picks single white primrose flowers and distils them, 'and that is good for the lightness of the head; and for bringing of the speech again, mingle therewith the like quantity of Rosemary flower water and Cowslip water ...'[38] Primroses and cowslips do have a sedative effect, so at least the speechlessness caused by fear might have been helped. Stroke victims, though, were probably less lucky.

Perhaps the old felt lucky in any case, for having survived so many accidents and fevers. Women could be thankful if they had safely got through the business of childbirth, and, in this century, so could anyone who had managed to become ancient in spite of war, plague or religious persecution. It was no wonder that so many receipts referred to God's help.

Troubled Heads

The head is subject to disease or injury like any other part of the body, and in the household books there are treatments for physical illness, accidents and pain. Lack of sleep was also unpleasant. These were comparatively straightforward. Other conditions such as lethargy, frenzy, melancholy and madness were more difficult to understand.

Violent and abnormal mental symptoms have always been puzzling. Is a mad person choosing strange behaviour on purpose? Has a demon taken possession of mind and body or is the individual a victim of witchcraft or even of God's displeasure? Perhaps there is something physically wrong with the brain? And most important of all, what can you do about it?

The irrational nature of madness perhaps encouraged people to suspect a supernatural cause. Robert Burton, who wrote *The Anatomy of Melancholy* during the first part of the century, thought that some madness might be a punishment inflicted by God, or come from possession by demons, the malice of the devil or, even worse, the power of the devil exercised through witches and magicians.

HUMOURS

Today there is still debate about the precise causes of some psychiatric illnesses, with some having a physical component of faulty brain chemistry. Similarly in the past, much melancholy and madness was seen to be the result of a faulty humour.

The writers of the household notebooks were pragmatic. Because a bad physical humour could cause difficult behaviour, it followed that difficult behaviour could often be treated by physical means, purging or rebalancing the humour concerned.

Normal black bile might become excessive, and result in jaundice, quartan ague, leprosy, scurvy or several kinds of madness. However, any humour could become abnormal, or dry up, when it was said to be 'adust', or be excessive, with different consequences. Dotage might be caused by a cold humour, for instance, but a hot brain, with hot animal spirits, caused violent madness.[1]

The brain was naturally cold, according to humoral theory, and associated with phlegm and moisture. It was a useful organ to cool the blood. (It was not until the second half of the century that Dr Thomas Willis began to demonstrate scientifically that the brain was the seat of thought, memory, and passion.[2]) It should not be too cold, however. If it was, lavender ointment was 'good for all diseases in the heade that proceede of colde.'[3] It was rubbed into the 'place where your greefe is', the temples, the noddle or crown and nape of the neck. Culpeper confirms that it is a hot herb, 'of especial use in pains of the head and brain which proceed from cold, apoplexy, falling-sickness, the dropsy, or sluggish malady ...'[4]

Of course, a physical injury might cause trouble. Mrs Corlyon is confident in her knowledge of 'The trewe cause whence many of the Paines of the heade do proceede, how to know those paines and the Reameadyes for them.'[5] Pain was the result of 'opening of the heade' caused by 'ouer much moisture beyng about the Braine. By a sodaine iumpe or fall: Or by vehement ryding or such like.' The jarring jump or hard riding might indeed have caused physical damage, but the moisture was more likely to be humoral.

She had a manoevre to check if the jaws could open wide, but if not you could press the skull together:

> ... puttinge your face betwixt your handes setting your thombes under the great skull Bone, that is behinde your eares, your fingars reaching vpp towardes the moulde of your heade. Gather your face

into your handes leaning [on a table] somewhat harde and squeasing
your face and the temples of your heade togeather, lett your fyngars
meete about your heade and this continue for the space of halfe
an hower at a tyme, vsing this to doe often so long as you shall
fynde occasion.

As you did this you had to use a lavender ointment to anoint the
head, and have a hot drink of milk and herbs, 'drinck of it as hott
as you can holding it in your mouthe that the ayre may assende into
your heade ... and Godwilling it will helpe.'

Another receipt deals with corrupt humours originating from an
alarming condition in the head: 'A Medecine to clense the Braine,
to helpe those that have a corrupt ayre at theire Noses and to clense
the Lunges of such grosse humors as ar distilled downe from the
putrified Heade.'[6]

You start by chewing rosemary leaves 'that the ayer may assend
into your head,' and then, bending down, 'voide the humours out of
your mouthe, as they do fall. Do this in the morninge fasting and two
howers before you goe to Supper for the space of halfe an hower at a
tyme', changing the rosemary leaves occasionally. Then eat a couple
of mouthfuls of shredded pennyroyal and hard honey, beaten together. When you have had enough of this, make 'tentes to putt vpp
into your Nose to open the conductes [conduits, passageways] and to
drawe down the corrupte matter that offendeth.' The tents were of
fine linen cloth, shaped like a narrow cone. They were dipped in the
juice of primrose leaves and a little clarified butter 'to make them to
slippe'. Put them up your nose and leave them there 'a pretty while:
then take them out, and wett them againe in the iuyce only' (no more
butter) and put them back. This was done for half an hour at a time,
and should be continued for 'a good space'. It sounds like an attempt
to clear blocked sinuses. Another simpler 'Comfortable Medecine for
paine in the Heade'[7] has similar tents put into the nostrils, this time
moistened with rose water and dipped into powdered nutmeg.

Another seventeenth-century complaint, hard to account for
today, unless satirically, is relieved by a receipt which confuses the
distinction between food and medicine in a poultice made from
edible ingredients, which would have been to hand in the kitchen:

A Medecine good for those that ar troubled with winde in their Heades[8]

Take a peece of sharpe leauen Doughe as bigg as an Aple and halfe an ownze of Comming seede fynelye beaten, worke it vpp in the doughe, and make it in a litle loofe then bake it vppon the hearth, and when it is well baked, open the loofe, and moisten the crumme a litle eyther with Malmesye or Aquavitae, then take two pretty peeces of the crumm, and putt them betwixt the foldes of a lynnen clothe and so fasten them somewhat warme to your eares, and lett them lye there for the space of twelve howers and then lay newe. This doe five or six tymes, and keepe your eares and your heade very warme both at the tyme and after, and it will helpe.

HEADACHE

Headaches and migraine are more familiar symptoms. Headaches were treated very often with an aromatic herbal plaster applied to the temples. Or the temples were rubbed with scented oil. Markham has a clutch of receipts of this kind, one for pads of dried rose-petals steeped in rose-water, camomile juice, woman's milk and vinegar, sprinkled with nutmeg.[9] This is very similar to a remedy for insomnia by Mrs Corlyon.[10] Others by Markham use oil of lilies, rue in vinegar, or a plaster of frankincense, doves' dung and wheat flour in equal parts.[11] In spite of all their knowledge of plants, seventeenth-century herbalists had not generally recognised the pain-killing property of willow-bark, which contains the fore-runner of aspirin.

Jane Sharp mentions a violent headache, sometimes one-sided, a feature of migraine, which she attributes to a distemper of the womb.[12] Modern women who suffer from migraine still sometimes notice a connection with pre-menstrual tension, and hormonal changes can provoke an attack.

An interesting suggestion for 'A Gargas or Medicine for the Meegreeme in the heade'[13] comes from Mrs Corlyon. It contains herbs in vinegar, plus mustard:

And then take a litle of it, as hott as you can suffer and holde it in your mouth as you shall feele occasion and then spitt it out, and take more and this doe five or six tymes euery morninge so long as you shall fynde occasion or feele your selfe greeued.

Migraine is still not entirely understood, but some headaches are caused by arteries at the base of the brain becoming temporarily swollen with blood. A hot mustard mix in the mouth might dilate the blood vessels there, and so possibly relieve pressure elsewhere.

SLEEP

A proper amount of sleep has always been considered necessary to good health. It was one of the six non-naturals (see p. 106):

It expels cares, pacifies the mind, refresheth the weary limbs after long work ... The chiefest thing in all physic, Paracelsus calls it, ... better than all the secret powers of precious stones and metals.[14]

Burton said it must be 'procured by nature or art, inward or outward medicines.' He has some sensible suggestions about external conditions – better to remove obstacles to natural sleep than to take remedies to cure insomnia. He recommends cultivating a tranquil mind, using a peaceful and quiet bedroom, clean bedlinen (perhaps he is hinting at the absence of bugs and fleas too), music, an agreeable book, darkness and the sound of running water, or silence.

A nightcap could be useful too. He quotes Andrew Boorde: 'a good draught of strong drink before one goes to bed', but himself recommends 'a nutmeg and ale, or a good draught of muscadine...' For those who wake in the middle of the night and cannot get back to sleep he suggests getting up and walking about a little until they feel cold, and then getting back to bed. Almost all this advice is still current today.

Nevertheless, some people might need more help than this. Herbal medicines can be especially effective. Mixtures of valerian, hops and passiflora are still sold over the counter to reduce stress and promote sleep. Lettuce is soporific, but there are two kinds used in herbalism, wild lettuce, *Lactuca virosa* which is a sedative,[15] and ordinary garden lettuce, *Lactuca sativa*, much weaker. Poppy, especially opium poppy, was frequently included in sleeping mixtures. Mrs Corlyon uses both:

An other Medecine to procure Sleepe[16]
Take of white Lettice Seede one ounze, and beate it in a morter, with a quantity of good white Sugar, vntill it do come to a moiste Conserue, and if you can gett it putt thereto halfe a spoonefull of Diacodyum then temper them togeather and keepe them so for your vse. And when you do take of it, eate a good quantity at a tyme and a pretty while after, drincke a draughte of Possett Ale, this doon dispose your selfe to reste, and you shall sleep.

A thirde Medecine to procure Sleepe[17]
Take of white Poppy Seede one spoonefull, beate it to powder then putt thereto a litle Possett Ale, made with Violettes Strawbery leaues and Cinquefoyle, drinck thereof warme and it will procure you to sleepe.

White poppies were probably opium poppies, *Papaver Somniferum*. Culpeper says that diacodium was a strong decoction of the seed-head boiled with sugar. The plant was cultivated in England but grew wild in Ireland. 'The syrup is a gentle narcotic, easing pain, and causing sleep; half an ounce is a full dose for an upgrown person, for younger it must be diminished accordingly.'[18] Poppy syrup was an ingredient of the gripe water for babies quoted on page 118. Diacodium could be bought from a druggist or apothecary for 3/4d per pound in 1676.[19] Culpeper goes on to explain that opium was obtained by drying the liquid collected after cutting the seed heads, but warned that this was 'very powerful, and, consequently, a very dangerous medicine in unskilful hands.'

FAILING MEMORY

Herbs might help to improve mental functioning. Markham has a useful receipt:

To quicken the wit.[20]
To quicken a mans wits, spirits, and memory; let him take *Langdebeefe*,
[ox-tongue, related to borage] which is gathered in *June* or *Iuly*, and
beating it in a cleene mortar; let him drinke the iuyce thereof with
warme water, and hee shall find the benefit.

Old age can weaken memory from a variety of causes too, such
as stroke and Alzheimer's in our terms. Gerarde suggests lily-of-
the valley as a help, though it should not be used without proper
advice today:

The flowers of the Valley Lillie distilled with wine, and drunke the
quantitie of a spoonefull, restoreth speech vnto those that haue the
dum palsie and that are fallen into the Apoplexie, & is good against
the gowte, and comforteth the hart.
The water aforesaid doth strengthen the memorie that is weak
and diminished, it helpeth also the inflammation of the eies, being
dropped thereinto.[21]

Agreeing with Shakespeare 'There's rosemary, that's for remem-
brance' Gerarde says that the flowers especially are good 'for al
infirmities of the head and braine proceeding of a colde and moist
cause; for they drie the braine, quicken the sences and memory, and
strengtheneth the sinewie parts.'[22]

MELANCHOLY

Melancholy was the prime example of mental anguish. The word
could describe something similar to our depression, but could also
include many other problems, for instance the misery of 'nuns,
widows and more ancient maids, ... enthusiasts, ecstatical and
demoniacal persons, ... love-melancholy, ... lycanthropia' and
religious mania.[23] It was difficult to distinguish between the categories, and overt madness was sometimes included. Robert Burton's
pioneering psychological and philosophical work, *The Anatomy of
Melancholy* goes into extensive detail over three volumes. Many

people were at risk from a variety of influences including the stars, climate, inherited predisposition, time of life, and above all corrupt or unbalanced humours:

> Such as have the Moon, Saturn, Mercury misaffected in their geni-tures; such as live in over-cold or over-hot climes; such as are born of melancholy parents; as offend in those six non-natural things [life-style factors, see p. 106], are black [i.e. with swarthy complex-ions, not people with naturally dark skin] or of a high sanguine complexion, that have little heads, that have a hot heart, moist brain, hot liver and cold stomach, have been long sick; such as are solitary by nature, great students, given to much contemplation, lead a life out of action, are most subject to melancholy. Of sexes both, but men more often; yet women misaffected are far more violent, and grievously troubled. Of seasons of the year, the autumn is most mel-ancholy. Of peculiar times: old age, from which natural melancholy is almost an inseparable accident ... [24]

The influence of stars was important to many practitioners, such as Nicholas Culpeper, but only traces of astrology appear in the household books. Here the cures were down to earth and logical. Get rid of the humour causing the trouble. To do this you could make broths, syrups, conserves or cordials. All the collections have receipts for this widespread condition.

Sometimes literal purging was prescribed, for instance in this Barrett receipt:

> A purging broath for mellancolly[25]
> Take a pint of broath where in mutton or Chicken hath been boyled, scum off the fat very clean, then take buridg flowers, bugloss flowers, rose mary flowers, St John wort flowers, red rose leaves, take of each of these as many as you can take up, betweene y[ou]r fingers. & twice as many currants as you can take up between y[ou]r fingers, & half a nutmeg sliced, seeth all these in y[ou]r broth half an hour, then take an ounce of the best scena & put it into the broth, & let it seethe one walme [come to the boil once], then take it off and cover it very close, and let it stand all night, in the morning straine out as much

as you can drinke at one draught, you must warme it luke warme &
then drink it, & lye in your bed an hour after you have taken it, and
fast three or foure hours.

These herbs are interesting. Like langdeboeuf mentioned above,
borage is a (modern) tonic for the adrenal glands, useful after stress.
Gerarde says that a syrup of the flowers 'comforteth the heart, purgeth melancholy, and quieteth the phrenticke or lunaticke person'.[26]
Viper's bugloss is a closely related plant. St John's wort has recently
been rediscovered as an anti-depressant, while rosemary is a nervine
stimulant. As for the roses, at this time 'leaves' seems to mean petals
rather than the green leaves of the plant, and were a very frequent
ingredient in all kinds of remedies. Senna pods are a powerful laxative. (If your depression was caused by constipation this would
certainly move you to cheerfulness, and the extra rest might have
helped as well.) Gerarde remarks of senna 'It voideth foorth fleg-
matike and cholerike humors, also grosse and melancholike, if it be
helped with some thing tending to that end.'[27]

Sometimes a herb was used in a modern way, simply because it
was good for the condition without reference to humour. Borage
again is the herb of choice:

> To comfort the heart, and take away Melancholy.[28]
> Take the juyce of Borage foure pound, the flowres of Borage halfe a
> pound: let these stand infused in hot embers fourteene houres, then
> being strained and clarified, put to of good Suger two pound, and
> boyle it to a sirrop.

The herb was mentioned by Gerarde too:

> Those of our time do vse the flowers in sallads, to exhilarate and
> make the minde glad. There be also many things made of them,
> vsed every where for the comfort of the hart, for the driuing away
> of sorrowe, and increasing the ioie of the minde.[29]

Mrs Corlyon also used rosemary. This was a syrup to be made in
summer, and kept for use later in the year:

A Syrupe or Conserue to open the Pipes to comfort the Harte and to expell Melancholye[30]

Take a quart of Honnye and putt it into a wide mouthed glasse add thereto so many of the flowers of Rosemarye as you can moisten therein by stirringe them well togeather, then sett it in the Sonn 2. or 3 dayes and as the Honny waxeth thynn with the heate of the Sonn, so stuffe it full with the flowers, this do so longe as there aryseth any moisture to couer the flowers, and when your Honny beynge thoroughly melted in the Sonn in this sorte will containe no more flowers, then beynge well stirred togeather, sett it in the Sonn to distill togeather the space of fower monethes, and it wilbe like a Conserue you must turne your glasse oftentymes that all sydes may take the Sonn alike And when you haue thus doen keep it for your vse. And when it is a quarter of an yeare olde take thereof euery morninge the quantity of a Wallnutt and you shall fynde the operation thereof to be very effectuall.

She also has a syrup which could be made for use at once if rosemary was available fresh, or dried in half the quantity. 'A very good drinck for those that be geuen [given] to Melancholy, and weepinge'.[31] A quart of claret and half a pound of sugar were brought to the boil and skimmed. A quart of rosemary flowers and half an ounce of cinnamon were added, then simmered for an hour. When cold you took a little with some more claret after meals and before going to bed.

A more elaborate cure for the Head family was to make a distilled medicine, more like a liqueur, which was no doubt cheering. The balm and cowslip used here are also soothing herbs. Going out into the garden to gather the flowers at their peak would have been a pleasant experience in itself. Fumes of melancholy are subtly different from a gross humour, perhaps marking a slight withdrawal from classical theory:

The Mallancholly Water[32]
Take of single stock jully flowers, or wall flowers foure handfulls, of Rose mary flowers 3 handfulls of damaske rose leaves 3 hand-fulls, of mary gold leaves 4 handfulls, of pinck flowers 4 handfulls;

of burradg flowers 2 handfulls of bugloss flowers 2 handfulls, of Cowslip flowers 4 handfulls; of Clove jully flowers 4 handfulls, of Balme leaves 2 handfulls; You must put these flowers as the time of the yeare will affoord them into a quart of [?]La Cannary Sacke, in a stone jugg close stopped, some times stirr the Sacke & flowers together, when all the flowers are infused, then add to it a quart of sack more, as alsoe these ingreedents following; half half [sic] an ounce of Cinomond grossly beaten, one ounce of anniseeds brused, 2 nutmegs sliced two penny worth of english safron, after all these things are well incorporated into the pottle of Sack, distill them all together in a cold still fast luted [sealed] with past[e], fasteing in the nose of the still, 2 graines of muske & one graine of amber greace, t[ha]t the distilled liquour may run through it into the Glass, distilling it with a soft fire, put in the glass into which it distills 6 ounces of white Sugar Candy finely beaten, then set your Glass one houre in hot water t[ha]t the sugar candy may well incorporat, take of this water 3 spoonfulls at a time in a morneing 3 times a week or oftener, it cures all mallancholly fumes, comforts the hearte & infinitly revives the Spiritts.

Yet there was also another kind of therapy based on pleasant company, music and agreeable surroundings, which had been advocated by the Renaissance humanist Marsilio Ficino. Advice given by this fifteenth-century Italian scholar, to avoid black bile, included looking often at shining water and bright green and red colours, with enjoyment of gardens and countryside. Strolling through pleasant meadows and travel on horseback or in carriages or sailing boats was commended. One should be occupied in varied non-demanding occupations, and have the companionship of cultivated friends.[33]

Burton cites many classical precedents for cheering the mind – music, 'mirth, and merry company,' as well as diversions such as singing, dancing, maskers and mummers. The senses should be recruited with agreeable smells, pleasant things to touch and taste, and pretty girls.[34] This was good advice in general, though perhaps it might be difficult to achieve if you were poor – and poverty was also a source of melancholy.

LETHARGY

We should consider lethargy to be a symptom of an underlying illness, as well as a component of depression, but the household books and herbals treat it as a disease in its own right. Markham has an extremely drastic way of dealing with it:

> For the lethargy[35]
> For the Letharge or extreame drowsinesse, you shall by all violent meanes, either of noises or other disturbances force perforce keepe the party from sleeping; and whensoever he calleth for drinke you shall giue him white wine and Isope water of each a like quantity mixt together, and not suffer him to sleep aboue foure hours in foure and twenty, til he come to his owne former wakefulnesse, which so soone as he hath recouered, you shal then forthwith purge his head with the iuice of Beetes squirted vp into his nostrels as is before shewed. [In the receipt for frenzy, below.]

A more humane wake-up remedy was applied by Gerarde externally. In his article on mustard, he says 'It is good against the falling sicknes, and such as haue the Lithargie, if it be laid plaistewise vpon the heade (after shauing) being tempered with figs.'[36]

MADNESS

Spectacular and violent madness had to be treated, if necessary with strong herbal drugs, but might be grouped together with quite different illnesses. Gerarde suggests black hellebore for example.[37] Also known as the Christmas rose, it is a poisonous narcotic. (You may notice, sadly, that epilepsy is often lumped together with other conditions which we now know have nothing to do with it at all):

> ... Blacke Hellebor purgeth downwards flegme, choler, and also blacke choler especially, and all melancholike humors, yet not without trouble and difficultie ... [It should be given only to robust and strong people.] ... A purgation of blacke Hellebor is good for mad and furious men, for melancholike, dull, and heauie [heavy] persons,

for those that are troubled with the falling sicknesse, for lepers, for them that are sicke of a quartaine ague, and briefly for all those that are troubled with blacke choler, and molested with melancholie.

Another hellebore made a violent cure for various 'cold' conditions, including frenzy:

> The roote of white Hellebor procureth vomite mightely, wherein consisteth his chiefe vertue, and by that meanes voideth all superfluous slime and naughtie humours. It is good against the falling sicknes, phrensies, sciatica, dropsies, poison, and against all colde diseases that be of hard curation, and will not yeeld to any gentle medicine ... [38]

However, it should be given only to country people, who were thought to be tough!

Perhaps equally dangerous was Markham's remedy. He recognised here that the condition could be caused by inflammation inside the skull:

> For the frenzie[39]
> For frenzie or inflamation of the calles of the braine you shal cause the iuice of Beets to bee with a serrindge [syringe] squirted up into the patients nostrels, which will purge and cleanse his head exceedingly; and then giue him to drinke posset ale, in which violet leaue [leaf] and lettice hath been boiled, and it wil sodainly bring him to a verie temperate mildenesse, and make the passion of frenzie forsake him.

If it was difficult to treat physical illness in the home, serious depression and madness must have been even more of a challenge. Perhaps an extended family or large household made caring for people with such conditions just about bearable. Yet of all the afflictions mentioned in the household books, the threatened loss of reason was perhaps one of the most terrible, the most feared. The anguish expressed by King Lear echoes still:

> O! let me not be mad, not mad, sweet heaven;
> Keep me in temper; I would not be mad!

Beauty, Cosmetics, Perfumes and Soap

John Evelyn made an entry in his diary on 11 May 1654: 'I now observed how the Women began to paint themselves, formerly a most ignominious thing, & used onely by prostitutes ...'[1] Even a moderate person disapproved of cosmetics. A more extreme Puritan ethic certainly did not encourage the pursuit of beauty for its own sake, especially not counterfeit or painted beauty. The manuscript books seem to be more concerned with health than vanity. Yet it was all right to treat 'infirmities of the face', especially if caused by humoral problems. According to Lady Mildmay:

> The defects of this part being most visible, justly deserveth the more diligent search of cure. They are either occasioned from things without us, as blasts and venomings ... Or within us, as the stopping and inflammation of the liver; the signs whereof is foul pimples or warts ... Or of the abundant putrefaction of blood and phlegm in the vessels whereof cometh the smallpox, the arch enemy of this masterpiece of nature.[2]

Thus health and beauty receipts do overlap. The printed books generally have more cosmetic entries, several for dyeing hair for instance. These would have attracted buyers of course, especially the frivolous females often condemned from the pulpit. This is true of *Delights for Ladies*, at the start of the century, *A Treasvrie of Hidden Secrets*, in 1637, and the many editions of *A Queen's Delight*, part of the *The Queen's Closet Opened*, later on. Besides specific receipts for beauty, Dr Stevens' Water, found almost everywhere, claims it will make one seem young, among many other benefits. (See p. 51.)

FAIR OF FACE

Marriage was important for young women, and to marry well – that is to a well-connected and well-heeled husband – was no doubt a good thing. It was desirable to be desirable. A young man on the lookout for a wife naturally wanted a healthy one. Clear skin was an obvious indicator. A face marred by smallpox, flaky skin called 'morphew', undue redness, pimples or even sunburn, was unattractive. The pox caused terrible damage too, so it was important to cure any sores that might be taken as a sign of this disease.

The Parker manuscript has a group of receipts for health and beauty. The first and second are for avoiding pock-marks:

a singular good medison that the small pox shall not be seene[3]
take a very fatt piece of beefe powdred [salted] and boyle it very well then take a good quantity of the fattest broth strayne it and put to it an indifferent quantity of red rose water and beat them well together a great while and when the pox begins to itch anoynt them 2. or 3. times a day with it untill they be cleane gon of and when the party is well let them take broath of leane powdred beefe and mingle it with white wine and so wash the face therewith and it shall bring it to a smoothnes as it was befor and by noe means keepe the throat or head too hott.

to dry up the pox
take a pint of creame and as much saffron as will make it of a deepe yallow and boyle them together a quarter of an houre and keepe it in a Glase and when the pox begins to wheale [heal] warme some of the oyntment in a saucer and anoynt them with a feather day and night till they be dryed

The principle seems to be to keep the skin soft with grease, either of beef fat or cream. Salt in the mixture would have been mildly disinfectant. White wine was astringent, so that the lesions would be encouraged to dry up. Saffron was mentioned by both Gerarde and Culpeper as being good for epidemic diseases such as smallpox, so perhaps external application would help as well.

The Kidders collected a considerably less attractive remedy:[4]

A water for the face after the small pox
Take a gallon of small white wine 8 pints of rosemary flowers 3 pints of sheld snails 3 limons sliced one handful of balme one handful of flax seed and foure sheets of venus [sic] paper and a welp of nine days ould, take the snailes and shell them and wash them in 12 waters and putt them into a linning cloath and drean them, then kill the dog and flea [flay] it, fling away the head and dry the foure quarters in a linin cloath until it be well dryed then putt them into a glas slided [?] together and drawe it with a quick fier the first pint will be principlle the 2nd and 3rd pritty good putt to each pint 2 ounces of white sugar candy finely beaten soe keep it in glasses and beath the face 2 or 3 times a day with a fine cloath or a tuff [tuft?] of white plane silk.
Author Mis Elizabeth Eltonhead

This is a distilled water. So far so good up to the flax seed. Snails should not cause any surprise by now. Venus paper is more puzzling. But sadly, this is not the only time a puppy was sacrificed to beauty. A receipt for a pomatum starts off 'Fat of a young Dog one pound'.[5] Perhaps there was a feeling that a young life-force was somehow extracted in this process, and would help regeneration. In 1664, Elizabeth Pepys used 'puppy dog water, being put upon it by a desire of my aunt Wight to get some for her, who hath a mind, unknown to her husband, to get some for her ugly face.'[6]

Three years later, Elizabeth was still taking beauty cures, this time with Samuel's approval. On 28 May she went with two companions to Woolwich, ready 'to gather May-dew to-morrow morning, which Mrs Turner hath taught her as the only thing in the world to wash her face with; and I am contented with it.'[7] It was said to be good 'For heat in the Face, and redness, and shining of the Nose.'[8] May dew was special. Sir Hugh Plat describes how to gather it, after a clear night, with a 'cleane and large sponge ... from sweet hearbs,

grasse or corne.' Sir Hugh's dew was strained into glasses and left in
the sun for most of the summer, covered with 'papers or parchment
prickt full of holes,' until it was white and clear. There must have
been a lot of it to start with if it were not to evaporate completely.
Dew from fennel and celandine was good for sore eyes, and it was
better than rosewater for preserving fruit and flowers.[9]

There were other ways to improve the complexion with salves
or washes, such as these from the Parker MS:[10]

> for heat in the face
> take marigold leaues [probably petals] bruise them and put them
> into creame and boyle them tell they be very thicke then put them
> in a cloath and hang it up and the juce will run from it like an oyle
> which save and put it in a pot and keep it all the year

> to make the face faire
> take betony flowers and seeth them in white wine with which wash
> your face if you drinke it it will make you have a sweet breath

Presumably drinking it was an alternative, not a recommendation
to drink the stuff after use. An earlier receipt might be the source
of this. It has the same ambiguity and similar wording except that
the herb is rosemary. It comes from *The Treasvrie of Hidden Secrets*.

> To make the face faire, and the breath sweet.[11]
> Take the flowers of Rosemary, and boyle them in white Wine: then
> wash your face with it, and use it for a drinke, and so shall you make
> your face faire, and your breath sweet.

The Treasvrie has a more downmarket feeling about it than the more
aristocratic *Delightes for Ladies* or the trilogy of *The Queen's Closet
Opened*. It claimed to be based on 'sundrie experiments, lately prac-
tised by men of great knowledge'. I wonder how many experiments
they had to conduct before they discovered the secret of this one
– but who could resist using it, when it had such a social cachet? It
sounds almost good enough to eat:

A water for the face, used by Gentlewomen.[12]

Take Goats milke two pound fine flower [flour] halfe a pecke, the whites of three Egges, and make it from paste to little loaves, and bake it, but not too much: then take more of the said Goates milke, and crumme of the crummes of your bread into it, let it steepe all night, and wipe your face with a drie cloth, and then wash your face with the said milke, and in using this, it will make the face shine as white as snow.

Another to make the face faire.[13]

Take the shearing of Scarlet, foure ounces, the whites of two new laid Egges, white wine two pound, Rosemary flowers, or Rosemary it selfe, and seethe it or still it, but if you seethe it scum it cleane, and when it is cold, use it, and it will make the skinne looke smooth.

The 'shearing of Scarlet' would be the fluff removed from scarlet cloth after weaving and before sale. Possibly the scarlet dye of the cloth made it an attractive pink.

The following receipt may refer to acne. 'Worms' were around a lot. They were a cause of dental caries for instance, so blackheads might also be thought of as little worms in the pores. Lady Mildmay has a receipt for a red face with pimples, which is also 'good for the little black spots which you call whay worms.'[14] The following comes again from the Kidders:

To Kill the Black wormes in the face[15]

Take 2 onces of night shade watter one once of red wine vinegar halfe an once of salt prunella and bathe the face 2 or 3 times a day with it probatum

Nightshade water seems rather like overkill, but it was for external application. 'Salt prunella' may possibly refer to self-heal, *Prunella vulgaris*, which has astringent and healing properties, as the popular name implies.

A sunburnt skin was all right for a man, leading an active life out of doors. But for women it was less admired. Ladies didn't do manual work in the fields, so if you had social pretentions you might need to bleach your skin. You might simply prefer to look pale in any case:

> A Water good for Sun burning.[16]
> Take Water drawn off the Vine dropping, the flowers of white Thorn, Bean-flowers, Water Lilly-flowers, Garden Lilly-flowers, Elder-flowers and Tansie-flowers. Althea-flowers, the whites of Eggs, French Barley.

> Another to remove high colour in the face.[17]
> Lemons laid in Buttermilke, is an excellent meanes to remove high colour in the face.

Freckles were undesirable as well, apparently even for men. Here sympathetic magic reinforces the herbal water, which must be used as the moon wanes. As it does so, the freckles fade away likewise. Or so it was hoped. The May connection existed here too, probably because elder leaves would be growing strongly then:

> To take away the freckles in the face.[18]
> Wash your face in the wane of the moone with a spunge, morninge and euening with the distilled water of Elder Leaues, letting the same drie into the skinne. Your water must be distilled in *Maie*. This is of a Trauailer [worker], who hath cured himselfe thereby.

Smooth Hands

'Trauailers' could also suffer from rough and stained hands. The next treatment is from *The Treasvrie of Hidden Secrets*. Its inclusion is possibly a clue to the intended readership. Salt with lemon is still a household remedy to remove stains nowadays, though it is a bit harsh on chapped skin.

> To make a water that taketh off all staining, dying and spots from the hands of Artificers, that get them by working, and maketh them white and faire. It is good for them that be Sun-burned.[19]

Take the juice of a Limmon, with a little Bay salt, and wash your hands with it, and let them drie of themselves: wash them againe, and you shall finde all the spots and staining gone. It is also very good against the scurffe or scabs.

Laundresses who washed clothes in the Great Wash, travelling from house to house to do this specialised work, probably suffered more than most from dried-out skin, especially in winter. Linen was soaked in a strong lye made of wood ash and urine, then rinsed (thoroughly, one hopes) and dried in the sun, if any. For them, and many others whose labour made them cold and wet, hand creams and lotions must have been more than welcome. Hand powder is not used today, as far as I know, but it was probably soothing and pleasantly scented:

To make smooth hands.[20]
To make an oyle which shall make the skinne of the hands very smooth: take Almonds and beate them to oyle, then take whole Cloues and put them both together into a glasse, and set in the sunne fiue or sixe daies; then straine it, and with the same anoint your hands every night when you goe to bed, and otherwise as you have conuenient leasure.

A Powder for the hands[21]
To a pound of Bitter Almonds take 2 ounces of Lupines & ye Peeles of 4 Oranges blanch the Almonds and Beate them as Small as may be adding nowe & then a spoonefull of rosewater to keepe them from oyling and the Lupines take ye Inward part of them and dry and Beate them searce them [sieve] and likewise the Orange Peele and when ye Almonds are dryed a little in the oven too [to] take the water out Grinde and Mix them with the Powder in a morter keepe them in a Gally pott

BAD HAIR DAYS

There may have been occasions when hair fell out after a fever. Sometimes, the head was shaved to apply poultices or other treatments. Men went bald, then as now. But the fashion for wigs meant that it wasn't much of a disadvantage for men to lack hair. Many, including Charles II, had it cropped or shaved on purpose. A wig had the advantage that it could be removed for delousing, though Pepys had a periwig supplied by his barber complete with nits.[22] For women, though, hair was an erotic symbol. There might be a need for receipts to make it grow. The Aqua Mellis mentioned in the following receipt was distilled honey, available from an apothecary if you didn't want to make it yourself:[23]

How to make Hair grow.[24]
Take half a pound of Aqua Mellis in the Spring time of the year, warm a little of it every Morning when you rise in a Sawcer, and tie a little spunge to a fine box comb, and dip it in the water, and therewith moisten the roots of the Hair in combing it, and it will grow long, thick, and curled in a very short time.

If honey by itself was not enough you could reinforce its effect with a little sympathetic magic.

To make Hair grow thick.[25]
Take three spoonfulls of Honey, and a good handful of Vine sprigs that twist like wire, and beat them well, and strain their juyce into the Honey, and anoynt the bald places therewith.

In Elizabethan England, fair or red hair was considered the most beautiful. The Queen herself had red hair, so it was obviously the best. There were dyes that could help if you wanted to be in fashion. William Turner said, with disapproval, that some used marigolds 'to make their hayre yelow ... not beynge content with the natural colour which God hath gyven them.'[26] If your hair was black it could be changed to 'a Chesnut colour' with oil of vitriol.[27] But 'you must doe it verie carefully not touching the skin.' Most definitely not. Vitriol is corrosive. However, by the middle of the seventeenth century, fair was not the only colour. *A Queens Delight* suggests using a silver groat or sixpence dissolved in aqua fortis – nitric acid – to dye beard or hair black[28] Perhaps it would be better to stick to yellow after all with a harmless receipt:

To make haire as yellow as gold.[29]
Take the rine or scrapings of Rubarbe and steep it in white wine or
in cleare lie [lye], and after you have washed your head with it, you
shall wet your haires with a spunge or some other cloth and let them
dry by the fire, or in the Sun. After this wet them, and dry them
againe, for the oftener they doe it, the fairer they will be, without
hurting your head any thing at all.

Shampoo, not to mention hair conditioner, purpose made for all
types of hair, is something we take absolutely for granted. But in the
receipt books I have found nothing specifically for simply making
hair clean. There are occasional references to washing it, for instance
as a preliminary to another receipt for yellow or golden colour by
Sir Hugh Plat.[30] Perhaps imported fine Castile soap was used. But
also perhaps, not very frequently. There might well be need for a
remedy for unwelcome colonists of the scalp.

For the wormes in Haire[31]
Wash your haire with flower of Brimstone & Vinegar mingled, & it
will kill the wormes./. Boyle a small handfull of the tops of century,
& two drams of juniper berries in five or 6. ounces of vinegar. Strain
it & adde six drams of hony; & bathe the part.

As with dental caries and blackheads, 'worms' seems to have been
the word for small and inconvenient causes of blemishes. Here they
are probably simply headlice or nits. Sulphur in brimstone and vinegar may well have got rid of them. The subsequent sweet-and-sour
lotion would have been sticky, but perhaps it was worth it.

Hygiene

It is understandable that personal hygiene has only a modest slot in
the books. In London and large towns, spring water had been brought
by conduit to the streets since the Middle Ages, and there were wells
too. Very few houses had piped water. This began to change when
the New River project was finished by Hugh Middleton in 1613.

Spring water from Hertfordshire flowed to an Islington reservoir, connected to rich houses in London. It cost about £1 6s 8d per annum to be connected, but the water was sometimes available for only a few days a week, when a domestic storage tank could be filled up. Alternatively professional water-carriers might bring a supply to the house from a public conduit, as they had in the past, but not everyone could afford the charge. For the rest of the population of London, and people in the country, nothing much had changed. Someone had to go out and fetch it. For cooking and medicinal use 'fair water' is specified very often, sometimes running water or spring water is needed.

If, today, we had to collect it in a bucket from a stream, well, or stand-pipe in the street, I expect we should rapidly lose our habit of a daily bath or shower and make do with washing the bits that showed, with a rub down of the rest from time to time. But hands were washed with water sometimes scented with lavender. Perfumes for the body and clothes, or to sweeten the air, were essential. Bad smells, both private and public caused by rubbish tips and sewage, had to be counteracted. This was not only civilised but important for health. Stinks and miasmas might be a source of illness in themselves. A particularly good example is the plague. To carry a strongly scented pomander was a precaution against catching it (see p. 94).

A kind of steam-bath could be taken, which would have conserved water. Sir Hugh Plat gives clear directions for 'A delicate stoue to sweat in.'[32] As he says, 'I know that many Gentlewomen as well for the cleering of their skins as cleansing of their bodies, do now and then delight to sweat.' A large brass pot was filled with sweet herbs and water. It was closely covered except for an exit pipe through which scented steam could escape into the bottom of a bathing tub when the pot was heated on a small charcoal fire. The gentlewoman sat in the bathing tub fitted with a false bottom drilled with holes so that the steam could rise around her. She left her head outside, but a sheet fastened round her neck kept in the warm scented vapour. She could stay there 'for a long time without fainting' but had to beware of a draughty room 'least any sodain cold should happen to offend you whilest your bodie is made open and porous to the aire.'

If Castile soap was not available or too expensive, you could make your own, and perfume it as well. Lye is an alkaline liquid, and combined with fatty acids it produces soap, more or less crude according to the precise ingredients and proportions. Here is a plain one, made partly from burned ash-wood:

To Make Good Soap[33]
First you must take half a strike of ashen ashes and a quart of lime. Then you must mingle both these together. Then you must fill a pan full of water and seethe them well. So done, you must take four pounds of beast's tallow, and put it into the lye, and seethe them together until it be hard.

A strike was a local measure of capacity, varying widely from place to place. Basic soap might be made more acceptable with added scent:

To make Muske Sope.[34]
Take strong lye made of Chalke, and six pound of stone Chalke, foure pound of Deeresuet, and put them in the lye in an earthen pot, and mingle it well, and keepe it the space of forty daies, and mingle and stirre it three or foure times a day, till halfe be consumed, and to that that remaineth seven or eight daies after, you must put a quarter of an ounce of muske, and when you have done so, you must also stirre it, and it will smell of muske.

Shakespeare's Coriolanus was contemptuous of the Roman citizens when he said:

Bid them wash their faces
And keep their teeth clean ...

But how would they have cleaned their teeth in his time? How would he have done so himself?

Although we take them for granted now, toothbrushes as we know them are only about 250 years old. Their precursor was a fibrous root or stem, beaten at one end until it became a little brush. Toothpicks must have been around for as long as food has stuck between the teeth, ranging from gold ones, custom-made, to any spare splinter of wood.

The simplest dentifrice was salt, rubbed over the teeth with a cloth or finger, but the household books have more elaborate ones. I'm not sure my dentist would approve of the following example, though. The honey contains sugar, and the vinegar acetic acid, neither of which are friendly to tooth enamel:

To keepe the teeth both white and sound.[35]
Take a quart of hony, as much Vinegar, and halfe so much white wine, boyle them together and wash your teeth therwith now and then.

'But if your teeth be verie scalie, let some expert barber first take off the scales with his instrument', though the lady shouldn't let the barber use *Aqua fortis*, in case she was 'forced to borrow a ranke of teeth to eate her dinner, unlesse her gums doe helpe her the better.' Other powders could be made based on scented orris root and powdered pumice, alabaster, brick or other abrasive agent, made into a paste and then into rolls to be rubbed on the teeth.

Air-fresheners have a long history. The preferred Elizabethan and Stuart scent was of roses in various combinations, though gilly-flower, lavender and others were also appreciated. Rosewater was a household staple for many purposes. Sir Hugh Plat has a quick receipt, good enough for everyday use:

A Speedy Distillation of Rosewater.[36]
Stampe the leaues [mash the petals], and first distill the iuice beeing expressed, and after distill the leaues, and so you shall dispatch more with one Still, than others do with three or foure stils. And this water is euerie way as medicinable as the other, seruing in all sirrups, decoctions, &c. sufficiently, but not altogether so pleasing in smell.

You could make little aromatic cakes of herbs to burn, or put perfume into a casting-bottle to sprinkle around. Small bags of dried sweet herbs were packed away with the linen, a custom which survives even today. (Clothes could be scented too, most especially gloves.) Here are a couple of specimen receipts, but there are very many more:

To make perfume cakes to burn[37]
Take one ounce of Beniamin [Benjamin] lay itt in Rose water one night then take Damaske Rose buds chip away the whites and rotten leaves [petals] and take of the best leaves two ounces and a quarter and putt the Beniamin to the Roses and beat them small till it comes to a past, then putt to itt 8 graynes of muske made in fair powder ... beat itt well after the Muske is in that itt may be thoroughe mixed putt to itt halfe an ownce of fine Barrel sugar to make them burne Soe make them up in little cakes and lay in Rose leaves in the bottom and on the top of ... cakes and when they are dry putt them up in a close box and keepe them.

King Edwards perfume[38]
Take twelve spoonfuls of right red Rose-water, the weight of six pence in fine powder of Sugar, and boil it on hot Embers and Coles softly, and the house will smell as though it were full of Roses; but your must burn the sweet Cypress wood before, to take away the gross air.

Armed with the family collection of receipts, or one of the printed books, a fastidious seventeenth-century woman could make a good attempt to keep clean and fair – or fairly clean by our standards. Although a healthy sheen on the face and smooth soft hands were not always possible, the good housewife could at least do her best to keep noxious vapours away from her family.

Magic, Superstition and Other Odd Ingredients

What is magic? It is a slippery word, and has meant vastly different things at different times. It has an uneasy relationship with religion and science, somewhere between faith and technology. In the Renaissance, Natural Magic was a rational system of enquiry, seeking to harness the power of nature. Some ideas carried through to the seventeenth century, like a cloud from which science proper would be precipitated later on. In any case, 'magic' and 'superstition' are terms commonly used by someone who does not share the belief-system of another culture. To those inside the system, such ideas seem normal.

In early modern times, for example, a few sceptics were questioning the existence of witchcraft, but many others accepted it as just one more hazard in a dangerous world. Some of the best minds of the time, Isaac Newton and Robert Boyle, for instance, regarded alchemy as a serious field of enquiry, though admittedly difficult. Astrology was still a respected discipline for many, including Nicholas Culpeper.

Then, too, the seventeenth century had a very strong tradition of Christianity, both Catholic and Protestant, which included literal belief in the devil and in miracles. The supernatural was not abnormal. Sympathetic magic, the idea of like curing like, 'a hair of the dog that bit you', was not a difficult concept. Folk cures and old beliefs persisted. If an amulet, ritual or spell was thought to help when you were ill, and most needed hope and comfort, it was in itself a medicine.

ANIMALS

It has already been pointed out that very many animals and animal parts were used in medicines. Horns, hoofs, skin, gall, stones from the stomach, the bone of a stag's heart, which was not a bone at all but cartilage,[1] fat from food animals, such as pigs, as well as from cats and dogs, foxes' lungs, poultry, fish-bones, eel skin – the list goes on and on. They are mostly by-products of farming, hunting, and fishing, and not wasted but put to use. Even non-vertebrates were exploited: (see p. 67) for some earthworm receipts, for example. Using such materials seems to be based on long tradition. Many of them can be found in Dioscorides, some as far back as Pliny. For instance, the receipts for snails, slugs, and earthworms show a clear trail back into the past.

It may be possible to divide the animal products into two categories. Firstly, the substance may be thought to act on the body in the same way as a herb or mineral. Snails are an example. The froth from a snail in woman's milk was a cure for fever in the Anglo-Saxon *Lacnunga* manuscript.[2] They slip into receipts of the thirteenth century, for instance in MS BL Sloane 146, where the juice of salted black snails – perhaps slugs – is a remedy for hot gout.[3]

A common medicine for consumption was based on snails, sometimes boiled in milk[4] (see p. 104). A snail could also be used to soothe sore eyes; 'take a snaile bruised shell and all, & wrapping the same in a fine linnen cloath, lay it on the eye, at night, going to bed.'[5]

There are also many receipts for 'Snail Water' for a variety of ailments. Mrs Corlyon has one for yellow jaundice, which involves roasting a peck of snails, and distilling them with ale.[6] (Snail water continued to be used, even into the eighteenth century, at St. Thomas's Hospital, London, for instance, but by then it was a medicine for venereal disease, and also included earthworms.[7])

Is this magic? The snail, being slimy, could perhaps soothe a cough or soreness. It was similar to phlegm, so might cure by sympathy. Or, there could even be a really curative substance present: on 10 November 2001 an article in *The Guardian* newspaper, concerning snails nibbling letters in country post-boxes, suggested that they were not all bad. Scientists were developing drugs for pain, epilepsy, depression and schizophrenia using hundreds of poisons from some kinds of snails.

LIFE FORCES

However, other animals seem to be exploited for their vital spirits, including heat, or for their symbolic qualities. Sometimes the disease is transferred into the animal. The Queen's plague cure, p. 98, which used chickens to draw out the 'poison' of the pestilence, is one example. Then there is the following, a treatment of last resort for a desperate condition. If you or a loved person is dying, and you have tried orthodox remedies and failed, there may seem no other option but to turn to atavistic magic, or a mixture of magic and precious ingredients:

> A raire watter, which hath restored severall out of deep consumptions[8]
> Take a red Cock, pluck him a live, then slit him down the back
> & take out all his entrells, cut him in quarters & bruse him in a
> mortar, then put him in a still with a pottle of Sack, & a quart of
> new red Cows milk, a pound of Currants, beaten, & a pound of
> reasons of the sun ston'd & beaten, of penney roiall, two handfulls,
> of wild time, roasmary, & burradg, one handful, one quart of red
> rose watter, of Hartshorn & China [root] of eatch one handfull,
> & past up y[ou]r still & still it with a soft fire D[r]up in the Glass
> where in it stills one pound of sugar candey, beaten, twelve pene-
> worth of Leafe Gold, 7 grains of musk, 10 graines of amber greece:
> 7 grains of unicornes=horne. 7: graines of beasor stone, & when the
> Watter is all still'd mix these ingreadents with it & use it Thus. Every
> morning fasting, & every eve[n]ing, when you goe to bed, take 4 or
> 5 spoonfulls of it warme, for a month together. This hath cured a
> man whome the Physitions had given over.

Plucking the cock alive was incredibly cruel. Maybe the idea was to get his vital spirits as fresh as possible. The bird was then pounded in a mortar, distilled with half a gallon of sack (see note on weights and measures, p. 7) – and the milk. A *red* cock and cow are specified, perhaps because the red colour suggested vitality. The raisins of the sun (distinguished from raisins of Corinth, now called currants), the herbs, rose-water and hartshorn were more standard ingredients. China-root came from an Asian plant related to sarsaparilla.

After distillation the exotic components were added. Twelve pence worth of leaf gold was an expensive amount. Musk and ambergris were also precious. (In 1676 they cost five shillings and twenty shillings per dram respectively. A labourer had wages of about £15, and a moderately well-off family had £40–£60 per year.[9])

Unicorn's horn has strong magical properties. In the Middle Ages and beyond, it appeared in the treasuries of princes and kings, used to test for poison in food among other things, and literally worth its weight in gold. The Chief Druggist to 'the late *French* King Lewis XIV', a Monsieur Pomet, wrote a book translated into English as *A Compleat History of Druggs*. The third edition was published in London in 1737. He said that Charles I was presented with a horn seven feet long, weighing thirteen pounds and shaped like a wax candle, 'suppos'd to be one of the greatest that ever was seen in the World'.[10] One very much like this is preserved today by the Society of Apothecaries of London, as a link with their past history. In the seventeenth century it was still associated with poison, but had become an antidote as well as a means of detection.

Perhaps it seems special (or strange) to us because we know that the animal was a mythical one. The beautiful horn with occult powers of protection has been romanticised on the one hand, and explained away on the other, as a tusk of the narwhal. (This was acknowledged by the mid-eighteenth century.[11])

Bezoar stones were found in the intestines of some ruminant animals, especially oriental goats, and like unicorn horn, were thought to be an antidote to poison. They could cost up to forty shillings an ounce.[12] Although of animal origin, they were often grouped with precious stones.

It seems therefore that there was a lurking suspicion that the 'deep consumption' was caused by poison, or at least a bit of magic might be a second line of defence. One can catch the frantic hope too that perhaps physicians might be proved wrong in a prognosis of doom.

Unicorn's horn appears elsewhere in the same notebook, too, though less spectacularly, in a remedy for worms. The horn was mixed with expensive mithridate, the compound used as an antidote to poison described earlier.

Falling-sickness or epilepsy has always seemed a strange disease, the fits coming apparently for no reason, the patient being normal between them. Hippocrates had said that the gods were not involved, but a touch of the uncanny clung to the sufferers, nevertheless. It is understandable that treatments were sometimes desperate, too. The next remedy, the nastiest I have come across, definitely suggests that the life-force of an animal is being absorbed from its blood:

> For the Falling Sickness approved upon persons of severall ages & sexes where of one lives now in St Johns Hospital in Canterbury in 1648[13]
>
> For a man take a she mole, & for a woman a he mole & setting by a good fire let the party put the moles Head in his mouth & biting it, sucke the blood out of the moles mouth as lively as it can, let the party set their right foot bare upon the mole, untill the blood hath don working in the body, in case it worke not the first or second time, try the third time with a third mole, & if it worke at any of the 3 tryalls with him, then the drink with Gods blessing will cure him

Then follows a recipe for a drink made from herbs and spices boiled in Muscadine. The cross-gender of the mole is interesting. Possibly, as with humoral theory, there is a muddled idea that imbalance in the body is at work, so a contrary ingredient needs to be introduced. Putting a bare foot on the dying or dead mole might suggest that the malign agent of disease was passing into the animal, away from the patient, and the magic number three was allowed for several attempts.

Similar folk-cures included the belief that moles' blood in white wine would cure epilepsy. One of Markham's receipts for the falling evil also uses moles of the opposite gender to the patient, caught in the mating season in spring.[14] The whole animal was dried, ground to powder and added to an early-morning and bedtime drink. But in another remedy he acknowledges that the falling sickness 'be seldome or neuer to be cured', though the patient might get some relief by eating 'berries of the hearbe *Asterion*' (not identifiable now) during a waning moon or when the moon was in Virgo. Even carrying the herb next to the bare skin might help 'though this medicine be somewhat doubtful'.[15]

Doctor Butler is quoted in several manuscripts, including Wellcome manuscript 774, Townsend. Many of his receipts seem to have had an infusion of sympathetic magic. Here in the Kidder manuscript the strength of an ox is being called on to build up a weak back with a nourishing caudle or soup:

Doctor Butlers Cawdle for the Back[16]

Take of the pith in the ox back Cleane picked halfe a pound beate itt small and grind itt well and a quarter of a pint of muscadine then straine itt and boyle itt with 6 Dates sliced 3 or 4 stickes of cinamon and as many of large mace put to it nutmeggs sliced 6 spoonfulls of red rose watter 4 onces of sugar lett all these boyle togather a little then take itt from the fyer and take this 2 or 3 days togather first and last put a little powder of Corall and amber to itt.

The Strange Case of the Unburied Skull

The human skull is a ghastly parody of the human face, with its rictus grin and blank eye-spaces. No wonder if it aroused awe, fear and respect in the past, and was one of the defining images of death (and hope of resurrection) in the Middle Ages. From these feelings it is only a small step to regard the skull as possessing some of the strength and qualities of its previous owner, which may be exploited for the benefit of the living. Besides, in Galenic medicine, and in Culpeper's view, the brain was regarded as the seat of the animal spirits, which included the five senses of seeing hearing, tasting, smelling and feeling, as well as internal senses of imagination, judgement, and memory.[17] Perhaps something of these animal spirits survived in the bone which had surrounded the brain. It had been a Renaissance belief, too, that because Man was the greatest of God's creations, his body parts were the most potent of all in medicine.

Whatever the rationale, however, human skulls formed part of the Renaissance pharmacopoeia, and persisted as an ingredient of medicine at least until the eighteenth century. Monsieur Pomet states that skulls were those of 'Criminals newly hang'd, stripp'd of the fleshy Membrane, and the Brains taken out, being well washed and dried ... is what the Druggists sell by the Name of Human Skull.'[18] The going price in London in 1676 was between eight and eleven shillings, 'if found'.[19]

Pomet remarks that:

> ... Man's Skull is a specifick Medicine in the Cure of the Falling-Sickness, and indeed of most Diseases of the Head, taking of the crude Powder, rasp'd from the fresh Bone of the Skull, one Scruple or two, in any proper spirituous Liquor. The Oil and volatile Salt are for the same Purposes, but in less Quantities.

In the household books, powdered skulls were indeed called for in treatments for epilepsy, and also for other afflictions such as palsy and loss of speech, which would now probably be attributed to Parkinson's disease or a stroke.

Here is Mrs Corlyon's recommended remedy:

> An especiall good Medecine for the fallinge Sicknesse[20]
> Take of the Skull of a mans heade and of Hepyonye rootes digged in the latter ende of Februarye of eche one ownze of Bettanye six drammes and of Lauander Spike 3. drammes The Skull muste be fyled very fyne and beaten very well in a morter. The rootes and Hearbes muste be dryed in the shadowe and then made into smale powder and all must be mingled well togeather.

Lady Mildmay had a more elaborate cordial which included conserves of anthos (rosemary flowers), betony, sage and cowslips, preserved citron peel, powdered afterbirth, powdered mistletoe, powder of man's skull calcined (strongly heated), peony roots, various preparations of balm, aromatic syrup and sweet oil of vitriol.[21] Both women advise taking note of astrological factors. Mrs Corylon remarks that the medicine is best taken 'in the beginning of the Springe, when the Sonn is new entered into the Signe Aries. Neverthelesse it hath had good successe at other tymes.' Lady Mildmay recommends a regime based on the 'full and change' of the moon.

The receipt given on p. 152 from Mrs Miller, for 'Palsey water, alsoe for Apoplexies or distempers or ffumes in the head' was also linked to the change of the moon. It too contained herbs, including calming lavender, and 'dead mens skulls in fine powder'.

The moss that grew on an unburied skull was as valuable a commodity as the skull itself. Culpeper claimed that 'Each moss partakes of the nature of the tree on which it grows, the oak is binding ...' so the moss on the skull must have partaken of the nature of the human bone. Pomet explained helpfully that (at least when he was writing) London druggists sold skulls with moss upon them. They had belonged to men who had died violently, and, he thought, the heads themselves sprouted the vegetation, in the same way that hair and beards apparently continue to grow after death.

This is a link with another group of even stranger medicines, the various sympathetic powders and ointments originating in the Renaissance if not before.

Wound Salve

I begin with Paracelsus (or possibly one of his followers), who explained that the power of 'Simpathy, or Compassion, hath a very great power to operate in humane things: As if you take Moss that groweth upon a Scull, or Bone of a dead body that hath lain in the Air' to make 'An admirable Oyntment for Wounds.'[22]

The ingredients of the ointment were the moss, 'Man's Grease', i.e. human fat, mummy, which purported to be from Egyptian tombs, man's blood, linseed oil, oil of roses and bole armeniac, a medicinal clay from Armenia. They were beaten together into an ointment, and kept in a box. If a person was wounded, a sliver of wood was dipped in his blood, dried, then pushed into the box of ointment and left there. Meanwhile, the wound was simply bandaged with new (clean) linen, and washed with the patient's own urine every morning:

After this manner, you may Cure any one that is wounded, though he be ten miles distant from you, if you have but his blood. It helpeth also other griefs, as the pain in the Teeth and other hurts, if you have a stick wet in the Blood, and thrust into the Oyntment, and there left. Also, if a Horses foot be pricked with a nail by a Farrier or Smith, touch a stick with the blood, and thrust it into the Box of Oyntment, and leave it there, it will Cure him. These are the wonderful Gifts of God, given for the use and health of man.

A weapon ointment was made in the same way, with the addition of some honey and ox-fat. This was used to anoint the weapon that had made the wound, to cure the injury without pain. 'But because the Weapons cannot alwayes be had, the Wood aforesaid is better.'

We have encountered Sir Kenelm Digby previously, with his nourishing broths. He was an adventurer, linguist, a member of the court of Queen Henrietta Maria in exile, one of the founder-members of The Royal Society. He also advocated the use of a 'sympathetic powder' of this kind. Some contemporaries were sceptical, but it has been pointed out that a simple dressing on the wound itself probably promoted healing better than a salve of dubious curative power.[23]

A similar receipt appears in the first section of *The Queen's Closet Opened*. Again, the wound is healed by sympathetic magic, though the compiler simply takes it at face value:

To cure any wound though the Patient be never so far off.[24]
Take a quart of pure Spring water, and put into it some Roman Vitriol, and let it dissolve, then if you have any bloud of the wound either in linnen or woollen, or silk, put the cloth so blouded in the water, and rub the cloth once a day, and if the wound be not mortal the bloud will out; if it be, it will not. Let the Patient keep his wound clean, washing it with white Wine; when ever you wash the cloth, the party wounded shall sensibly finde ease: let the cloth be constantly in the water.

It is interesting to see that an element of prognosis has crept in here. It is a means of foretelling whether the patient will live or die, and a cure is not guaranteed, in spite of the optimism of the heading.

BIRTH MAGIC

The act of producing another human being has always seemed full of wonder. Even today, in spite of all our biological knowledge, childbirth still evokes awe. It is therefore not surprising to find that there are many superstitions associated with giving birth. Some of these were mentioned in Chapter 8, but a few more can be added here.

In the seventeenth century, and earlier, a pregnant woman had to be careful about what she looked at or imagined. The power of suggestion could work for good or ill. Robert Burton tells the story of an ugly man with an ugly wife, who 'hung the fairest pictures he could buy for money in his chamber,' so that their children would be beautiful. Yet, if a pregnant woman saw horrible sights, or even imagined them, her child could be born deformed. Cravings were dangerous, too. 'Great-bellied women, when they long, yield prodigious examples of this kind, as moles, warts, scars, harelips, monsters ...'[25]

Jane Sharp thought that conception during menstruation could result in a monster, 'mole' or moon-calf (a grossly deformed foetus), 'a mishapen piece of flesh without figure or order.'[26] It is sad to think that women could be blamed for something we would think of today as tragic pathology.

Barrenness might be caused by natural factors, but also by enchantment 'when a man cannot lye with his wife by reason of some charm that hath disabled him'. In this case Jane Sharp suggested a French counter-spell: 'to piss through his wives Wedding ring and not to spill a drop ... Let him try it that pleaseth.'[27]

More happily, eagle stones were an almost infallible way to prevent miscarriage and ensure an easy birth. The stone was hollow, with another little stone inside it, an obvious parallel with a womb containing a child. An intrepid climber had made his way to an eagle's nest on a mountain to steal it away. Hence the name. It acted like a magnet. Tied to the mother's arm it prevented premature labour, but when the proper time came, 'The Eagle stone held to the secrets, draws out both Child and *Secundine* [afterbirth],' said Jane Sharp. You had to be cautious at this point however: 'hold it to no longer for it will draw forth Womb and all ...'[28]

Sympathetic magic is certainly invoked in this remedy to increase mother's milk:

> Some say that by sympathy a Cows Udder dried in an oven, first cut into pieces, and then powdered, half a pound of this powder to an ounce of Anniseed, and as much of sweet Fennel-seed, with two ounces of Cummin seed, and four ounces of Sugar, will make milk increase exceedingly: ... some prescribe the hoof of a Cows forefeet dried and powdered, and a dram taken every morning in Ale; I think it should be the hoofs of the hinder feet, for they stand nearest the Udder, where milk is bred. I mislike not the experiment, but our Ladies thistle is by Signature [i.e.the Doctrine of Signatures], and (the white milky veins it hath) well known to be a very good help to women that want [lack] milk.[29]

DUNG AND URINE

Of all animal products, dung and urine seem the least likely to be justified as therapeutic. There is generally an instinctive feeling of disgust about excreta. How did they ever come to be used? Roy Porter suggests that the idea may have originated in very archaic times, when disease was thought to be caused by demons invading the body. *Drekapotheke* (filth pharmacy) was an attempt to drive them out with revolting medicines using excrement and other disgusting things such as poisonous insects and so on.[30] This does make sense of a kind, but it means that the tradition, once established, persisted in spite of experience and commonsense, for a very long time indeed. Alternatively, the idea might have been rediscovered from copies and translations of classical texts.

It seems certain that excreta were in fact used. Pliny mentions dung as medicine, but with some scepticism. He has a fairly good opinion of human urine though, especially for eye complaints.[31] Dioscorides has hot cow-dung as a fomentation for sciatica (as in Mrs Corlyon's remedy for gout on p. 146), and goats' 'berries' in wine for jaundice.[32]

Here is almost the same receipt from Markham, although he uses the dung of sheep instead of goats and ale instead of wine:

For a desperate yellow Iaundisse[33]
For the yellow Iaundisse which is desperat and almost past cure; take
Sheepes dung new made and put it into a cup of Beare or Ale, and
close the cuppe fast and let it stand so all night, and in the morning take
a draught of the cleerest of the drinke, and giue it to the sicke partie.

Dioscorides lists the uses of the droppings of cows/bulls, goats,
sheep, wild swine, asses, horses, 'grass eaters', doves, poultry, storks,
vultures, mice, dogs and men. Plus that of 'earth crocodiles' for
making women's faces shine! The Anglo-Saxon leechbooks were
more selective, listing the dung of pigs, pigeons, goats, sheep, horses
and geese.[34]

Medieval receipts were fairly sparing too, though droppings
from farm animals and poultry make their appearance.

Horse-dung was used in alchemy and distillation as a source of
even, gentle heat. Soaking in a tub of hot horse dung, urine and
herbs, as in Kidder's receipt for the gout in arms and legs, given on
p. 145, was reasonable in its way. Steady warmth was applied to the
legs. Urine had been recommended as far back as Pliny as a cure for
gout among other applications.[35] (All the same it must have been a
relief to know that you didn't have to sit in the mixture up to your
neck in order to ease the pain in your arms.)

This one comes with a personal recommendation, from the
Townsend manuscript:

An excellent bath for swellinge in the legges[36]
take a hanfull of chickweede a handfull of comon mallowes an as
much red sage boyle these in a chamber lye [urine from chamber
pot] an bathe your legges when you goe to bed every night till they
are well this I know to be rare myselfe Sume doe put salt in it which
is very good.

Urine was also recommended to wash out an animal-bite or new
cut, both by Pliny and by Paracelsus in the wound salve mentioned
above, so it is not surprising to find the practice continuing 'To cure
the bite of a Dog, or a cut just doune' when the wound was washed
with chamber lye.[37]

It is an ingredient 'To restore Sight, tho lost' by H.S in the Barrett manuscript.[38] This is one of a section of at least twenty-four receipts on eye problems, which seem to have been common, or at least very worrying. It is similar to the receipt in the Parker manuscript, given on p. 80:

> Take smallage, rewe, fennell, vervine, egrimony Bettony Scabies [scabious] Autre [or] hound-tongue Eye-brite, pippernell & Sage of each of them a bout a handfull, distill all these together with the urine of a man Child which sucketh, a bout a pint with as much womans milk & 2 spoonfulls of english Honey & .5. graines of frank-encence, being thus distilled drop a drop or 2 into the eyes morning & evening H.S.

Possibly the baby's urine, and the nursing mother's milk, were thought of as agents for renewal. Even so, collecting a whole pint at a time might have been difficult. (But eyebright, as its name suggests, is a well-known practical remedy, even today, for inflammation in the eye.)

Doubts about this kind of medicine were starting to stir in the seventeenth century, though. Culpeper, to his credit, did not translate the dirty Latin bits from the *Pharmacopoeia Londinensis*. Instead, he took the opportunity to be very rude about the College of Physicians.

> As for Excrements there the Colledg makes shitten work and paddle in the turds like Jakes Farmers, I will let them alone for fear the more I stir them the more they stink.

Amulets, Talismans, Spells

This kind of magic did seem to be waning as far as the household books were concerned, though vestiges remained. Talismans and amulets had been carried or worn since very early times. Talismans are positive, thought to attract good luck or healing, whereas amulets are defensive, worn to avert dangers. They are still used today:

many people prize a special lucky coin or ring. They do make a few appearances in the household books, as for instance Doctor Butler's amulet 'for the mother and fainting' using dried fox testicles hung in a little bag near the navel (p. 131).

Another example was this addition to *The Queen's Closet* in the second edition:

> To cure the Tooth-Ache[39]
> The tooth of a dead man carried about a man, presently [immediately] suppresses the pains of the teeth.

In fact the teeth and claws of various animals were mounted in metal such as gold or silver so they could be hung round the neck or be worn as a ring. A piece of coral on a string was frequently given to babies. Perhaps its purpose was like a modern teething ring, to give the baby something hard to bite on when milk teeth were erupting, or perhaps it had magical protective powers. Red coral was also taken internally to preserve health, and to prevent convulsions in babies.[40] Culpeper said that it 'helps [that is, defends against] witchcraft being carried about one.'

Seashells or pieces of ivory could be used as talismans/amulets. The British Museum holds an interesting collection of such objects, including a toadstone ring with a gap in the mount, so that the magic is close to the skin. The toadstone was said to be extracted from the head of an old toad, but was in fact much less romantic. It was a fossilised fish eye. It was believed that it 'helps the bitings of venemous beasts, and quickly draws all the poyson to it, it is known to be a true one by this, hold it neer to any Toad, and she will make proffer to take it away from you, if it be right, else not.'[41]

Finally, I must mention an outright spell, reminiscent of an Anglo-Saxon health charm. It is written sideways in the Kidder manuscript, in the larger, less literate hand that alternates with a more educated one. This is the same hand as that of 'Capt Kidder his Recept' for urinary gravel. Whether there is any significance in writing it sideways on I cannot say, but it is the only one written thus in the manuscript:

a cure for the ague[42]
when the Ieues [Jews] led Christ to the please [place] of exsecutyon
they said he had a feauer [fever] butt he answered he had neither
ague, nor feauer and whoeuer did were [sic] these words written
aboutt there writte arme should neuer have ague nor feauer

No Expense Spared: Precious Stones, Pearls, Gold and Silver

The use of precious stones and metals in medicine is at the opposite end of the pharmacopoeia from dung and urine, but it has
an equally long history. Gemstones are mentioned by Dioscorides,
Pliny, in medieval lapidaries and Renaissance magical treatises.
They are of course rare, expensive and prized for their beauty, even
today. They were (and still are) associated with astrology, and were
sometimes thought to receive their power from the stars' influence.
In Paracelsan theory, metals at least were quasi-living things:

> ... No-man ... can teach that Metals are dead Substances, or do
> want life; seeing their oyls, salt, sulphur, and quintessence are the
> greatest Preservatives, and have the greatest strength and virtue to
> restore and preserve the life of man, before all other Simples, as we
> shall teach in all our Remedies assigned thereunto: Certainly if they
> had not life, how could they help Diseases, and restore the decayed
> Members of the Body, by putting life, and stirring up corporal veg-
> etation in them: as in Contractures, the Stone, Small-pox, Dropsie,
> Falling-sickness, Phrenzy, Gout, and several other Diseases, which
> for brevities sake I omit to mention. Therefore I say, That Metals,
> Stones, Roots, Herbs and all other Fruits have life in them, though
> of divers kinds, according to their Creation and growth, and the due
> observation of the time contingent thereunto.[43]

Not only mineral stones were valued. Some were of questionable
origin, such as the snakestone obtained from a serpent, or the toadstone extracted from a toad, in theory. Bezoar stones were real,
being found in the stomachs of some ruminants, and crop up, so

to speak, in many of the household and official remedies, as we have seen.

A cordial powder to 'stay the greatest vomiting and lose-ness what ever' in the Barrett manuscript contained the precious ingredients of unicorn's horn, bezoar stone, hartshorn, white and red coral, pearl, ivory, citron peel and exotic herbs, musk and gold. This has a Renaissance magic air, such as would not disgrace a guest at one of the Borgia's feasts.[44]

Gold was the most prized metal, being incorruptible for practical purposes. It had the symbolic quality of perfection, and was the most highly developed, to which other metals aspired, according to the alchemists. It was regarded as strengthening the heart, and associated with the sun and its life-giving power. Silver was also highly thought of, but was of a feminine nature, linked with the moon.

Culpeper's translation of the *Pharmacopoeia Londinensis* includes a list of the virtues of many precious stones, as well as several receipts containing powdered gemstones. These are mixed with herbs and other precious ingredients. Here are a pair of them, one 'cold' and one 'hot', to be administered to cure the contrary excess. A 'species' was a powder, here prepared ready to be mixed with a syrup to make up an electuary:

Species Electuarii de Gemmis frigidi[45]
Take of Pearls prepared three drachms; Spodium, Ivory, both sorts of Corral, of each two drams; the flowers of red Roses a drachm and an half; Jacinth, Saphire, Emerald, Sardine, Granate, Sanders white red and yellow, the flowers of Borrage and Bugloss, the seeds of Sorrel and Bazil, both sorts of Been (for want of them, the roots of Avens and Tormentil) of each one drachm; Bone of a Stags heart half a drachm: Leaves of Gold and silver of each fifteen: make of them all a Pouder according to art, and let it be diligently kept.
Species Electuarii de Gemmis Calidi *Merue*
Take of Troches Diarhodon, Wood of Aloes, of each five drams; white Pearl, Zedoary, *Doronicum*, Citron pils, Mace, the seeds of Bazil, Ambergreese, of each two drams; red Corral, white Amber, Ivory, of each five scruples: Saphire, Jacinth, Sardine, Granate,

Emerald, Cinnamon, Galinga, *Zurumbet*, [marginal note, Round Zedoary] of each one drachm and an half; Been, of both sorts, or instead of them the roots of Avens and Tormentil, Cloves, Ginger, Long Pepper, Indian Spicknard, Saffron, Cardamoms the greater, of each one drachm; leaves of Gold and Silver, of each two scruples, Musk half a drachm: make them all into a Pouder, and keep them close stopped from the air.

He goes on to comment:

The truth is, both these pouders are of too heavy a prise for a vulgar mans purse. They help afflictions of the heart, stomach, brain and liver, vain fears, melancholly, tremblings of the heart, and faintings, they help digestion, and take away sadness, and because the latter seems to be something hotter than the former, though neither of them exceed in heat or coldness: if you find the body afflicted by cold, you may give the hotter, if feaverish, the cooler. You may take half a drachm at a time in any cordial water.

Pearls were prepared by grinding them in a steel mortar, moistening them with rosewater so that the fine dust did not blow away. 'In the like manner is Corral and other precious stones prepared.'[46] Pearls were a tonic for the heart, increased the milk of nursing mothers, and helped consumption.[47]

Another equally costly medicine was:

Confectio de Hyacintho.[48]
Take of Jacinth, red Corral, Bole Armenick, Earth of Lemnos [marginal note, Terra Sigillata] of each half an ounce, the berries of Kermes, the roots of Tormentil and Dictamni, Citron seeds husked, the seeds of Sorrel, Purslain Saffron, Mirrh, red Roses, all the sorts of Sanders, bone of a Stags heart, Harts horn, Ivory, of each four scruples, Saphire, Emerald Topas, Pearls, raw Silk, the leaveas [sic] of Gold and Silver, of each two scruples, Camphire, Musk, Ambergreese, of each five grains with syrup of Lemmons make them into a Confection according to art.

He goes on to add: 'It is a great cordial, and cool, exceeding good in accute feavers, and Pestilences, it mightily strengtheneth and cherisheth the heart. Never above half a dram is given at a time, very seldom so much, not because of its offensiveness, I suppose its chargableness.'

The French druggist Pomet gives an almost identical receipt, but advises that musk and ambergris should not be included except on the advice of a physician, because it is women who use the confection most.[49] Musk and ambergris were 'very improper for the Sex, especially in any hysterical Case.' Both were used in perfumes, and perhaps were 'improper' because they had sexual undertones. He also explained that the bone of a stag's heart was not bone, but gristle.

A few individual qualities of some the mineral stones, according to the *Directory*, were said to be as follows:[50]

> *Jacinth or hyacinth*, strengthened the heart. *Emerald*, when worn resisted lust, helped falling-sickness and vertigo, took away foolish fears, folly and anger, and if it did this when carried on the person, 'beaten into pouder and taken inwardly, it will do it much more.' *Sapphire* resisted 'Necromantick apparitions', was an antidote to venomous bites and ulcers in the guts. *Granite* was good for the heart but bad for the brains, causing anger and insomnia. *Topaz* reduced inflammation (and would possibly even cool boiling water).

These were precious medicines indeed, not for the ordinary housewife such as Markham's to prepare, but probably to be bought at the apothecary's. Did they really do anything for the sick? By the eighteenth century, Pomet was doubtful. 'I am of Opinion with those who allow no other Virtue in all the precious Stones, than to absorb Acids.'[51] Earlier, in 1663, Robert Boyle was less sure:

> I am not altogether of their mind that absolutely reject the internal use of Leaf Gold, Rubies, Saphyrs, Emeralds, and other Gems, as things that are unconquerable by the heat of the Stomach. I think that in Prescriptions made for the poorer sort of Patients, a Physician may well substitute cheaper ingredients in the place of

these precious ones, whose Virtues are not so unquestionable as their dearnesse.[52]

Perhaps one should keep some openness of mind about all the receipts quoted in this book. Many of the herbal mixtures would have been useful, but others do appear unlikely to have cured serious diseases as claimed. Yet, in their day, they were accepted as good practice, studied, copied, recopied, and presumably swallowed or applied with as much hope as we, in our time, go off to the chemist to get our prescriptions made up. The human body is inclined, after all, to repair itself when it can. A very perceptive explanation was given by Richard Burton. He came close to the modern recognition of the placebo effect, the power of suggestion working through imagination:

> We see commonly the toothache, gout, falling sickness, biting of a mad dog, and many such maladies cured by spells, words, characters, and charms, and many green wounds by that now so much used *unguentum armarium* [weapon salve] magnetically cured ... All the world knows there is no virtue in such charms or cures, but a strong conceit and opinion alone ... The like we may say of our magical effects, superstitious cures, and such as are done by mountebanks and wizards ... An empiric oftentimes, and a silly [humble] chirurgeon, doth more strange cures than a rational physician.[53]

Perhaps every medicine was precious in its way?

Notes

Many manuscripts have been paginated, so I follow the page numbers as they appear. Otherwise folio numbers are given.

CHAPTER 1: THE STUART HOUSEEWIFE AND HOUSEHOLD BOOKS

1   Gervase Markham, *Countrey Contentments, The second Booke called the English Hous-wife*. Amsterdam & New York: Da Capo Press, Theatrum Orbis Terrarum Ltd. 1973. (Facsimile of edition published in London 1615), pp.1–4.
2   Sir Hugh Plat, *Delightes for Ladies*. London: Crosby Lockwood, 1948, from edition originally published 1609, p. 27.
3   Andrew Wear, *Knowledge & Practice in English Medicine, 1550–1680*. Cambridge: Cambridge University Press, 2000, p. 12.
4   Wellcome MS 3107, Edward & Katherine Kidder, about 1699, pp. 225–231, 209–211.
5   Jennifer K. Stine, *Opening Closets. The Discovery of Household Medicine in Early Modern England*. (Unpublished Ph.D. Dissertation, Wellcome Library), 1996, p. 145.
6   Wellcome MS 3107, Kidder, 1699, p. 185.
7   Markham, *The English Hous-wife*, 1615, p. 4.
8   Wellcome MS 1071, Barrett, p. 67.
9   Wellcome MS 213, Corlyon, pp. 53, 91, 317.
10 Markham, *The English Hous-wife*, 1615 and 1631 edition, p. 58.
11 Wellcome MS 1071, Barrett, pp. 27 and 38.
12 Wellcome MS 3769, Parker, f. 69 r.
13 Wellcome MS 213, Corlyon, p. 290.
14 W. M., *The Queen's Closet Opened, [Part 1] The Pearl of Practice*. London: Nathaniel Brook, 1655, p. 150.

CHAPTER 2: BACKGROUND TO 17TH CENTURY MEDICINE

1   Robert Burton, *Anatomy of Melancholy*. London: J. M. Dent, 1932, vol. 2, p.6. Originally published 1621.

2   Roy Porter, *The Greatest Benefit to Mankind: A Medical History of Humanity from Antiquity to the Present*. London: HarperCollins, 1997, p. 56.

3   *ibid.*, pp. 62–3.

4   Stephen Pollington, *Leechcraft: Early English Charms, Plant Lore, and Healing*. Norfolk: Anglo-Saxon Books, 2000.

5   *ibid.*, p. 453.

6   Gideon Harvey, *The Family Physician*. London: printed for T. R., 1676. Introduction, A4.

7   Marcilio Ficino, *The Book of Life*. A Translation by Charles Boer of *Liber de Vita* (or *De Vita Triplici*). Texas: Spring Publications, 1980.

8   Wellcome MS 213, Corlyon, p. 291.

9   Nicholas Culpeper, *A Physical Directory*, Or a Translation of the Dispensatory Made by the Colledge of Physitians of London. 2nd ed. London: Peter Cole, 1650. Directions, C verso.

10 Susan Mary Drury, *Plant Lore in England 1600–1800*. Unpublished M. Phil Thesis, Institute of Folklife Studies, School of English, University of Leeds, 1984. Also the following.

11 David E Allen & Gabrielle Hatfield, *Medicinal Plants in Folk Tradition: An Enthnobotany of Britain & Ireland*. Portland Oregon and Cambridge: Timber Press, 2004, p. 16.

12 Cited in Graeme Tobyn, *Culpeper's Medicine*. Shaftesbury: Element, 1997, p. 9.

13 Walter George Bell, *The Great Plague in London*. London: Folio Society, 2001, p. 202.

14 Cited in Liza Picard, *Restoration London*. London: Weidenfeld & Nicolson, 1997, p. 3.

CHAPTER 3: HERBAL MEDICINE

1   Wellcome MS 1071, Barrett, p. 18.

2   Gabrielle Hatfield, *Memory, Wisdom and Healing: The History of Domestic Plant Medicine*. Stroud: Sutton, 1999, p. 8.

3   Nicholas Culpeper, *The English Physitian*. London: Peter Cole, 1652, A5 v.

4   John Gerarde, *The Herball or Generall Historie of Plantes*. London: John Norton, 1597, p. 457.

5   *Culpeper's Complete Herbal*, London: Foulsham, n.d. p. 372.

6   Wellcome MS 3107, Kidder, p. 267.

7   Wellcome MS 213, Corlyon, p. 158.

8   Mrs M. Grieve, *A Modern Herbal*. Harmondsworth: Penguin Books, 1976, p. 426. Culpeper says much the same, though he adds a little sugar. *Culpeper's Complete Herbal*, p. 200.

9   Wellcome MS 1071, Barrett, p. 67.

10 *Gerard's Herball, The essence thereof distilled by* Marcus Woodward. London: Bracken Books, n.d. p. 42.

11   Gabrielle Hatfield, *Country Remedies*. Woodbridge: The Boydell Press, 1994, p. 23.

12   Harvey, *The Family Physician and the House Apothecary*, p. 36.

13   Culpeper, *A Physical Directory*, p. 80.

14   Harvey, *The Family Physician*, p. 6.

15   Wellcome MS 1071, Barrett, p. 27.

16   W. M., *The Compleat Cook and A Queen's Delight* (Facsimile reprint 1655). London: Prospect Books, 1984. *A Queen's Delight*, p. 88.

17   Wellcome MS 213, Corlyon, p. 243.

18   Wellcome MS 3107, Kidder, p. 23.

19   Plat, *Delightes for Ladies*, p. 59.

20   Wellcome MS 1071, Barrett, p. 27.

21   John Partridge, *The Treasvrie of Hidden Secrets*. London: Richard Oulton, 1637, Chap. 105.

22   This cookery book has been republished recently, edited by Anne Ahmed, wife of the present Master, as *A Proper Newe Booke of Cokerye*. Cambridge: Corpus Christi College, 2002.

23   Wellcome MS 1071, Barrett, p. 63.

24   Cited in Michael White, *Isaac Newton The Last Sorcerer*. London: Fourth Estate, 1997, p. 132.

25   *Everybody's Pepys*, edited by O. F. Morshead. London: G. Bell & Sons 1945, p. 238.

26   Gerarde, *The Herball*, p. 1070 onwards.

27   In 1676, mithridate cost six shillings a pound, according to Gideon Harvey.

28   Culpeper, *A Physical Directory*, p. 125.

29   *ibid.*, pp. 127–128.

30   *ibid.*, p. 173.

31   *ibid.*, p. 128. Gideon Harvey's price for this was two shillings a pound.

CHAPTER 4: ACCIDENTS AND EMERGENCIES

1   Culpeper, *A Physical Directory*, p. 72.

2   Pollington, *Leechcraft: Early English Charms, Plant Lore, and Healing*.

3   Cited in *Medical Works of the Fourteenth Century*, edited by the Rev. Prof. G. Henslow. London: Chapman and Hall, 1899, p. 90. From Harleian MS 2378.

4   Many aspects of medieval medicine are contained in the *Reports into Researches into the Medieval Hospital at Soutra*, Nos. 1–6, by Dr Brian Moffat and others. Edinburgh: SHARP Project, 1986 on.

5   *Leaves from Gerard's Herbal*, edited by Marcus Woodward. London: Gerald Howe, 1931, p. 105.

6   Culpeper, *A Physical Directory*, p. 126.

7   *Gerard's Herball*, ed. Woodward, p. 85.

8   Gervase Markham, *A Way to get Wealth* ... [Book 3] *The office of the Housewife*, London: Nicholas Okes for John Harrison, 1631, p.55. [Referenced after this as Markham, *The English Hous-wife*, 1631.]

9   Culpeper, *A Physical Directory*, p. 202.
10 Markham, *The English Hous-wife*, 1631, p. 18.
11 Wellcome MS 213, Corlyon, p. 300.
12 Wellcome MS 3547, Miller, f. 64 r.
13 Wellcome MS 3107, Kidder, p. 269.
14 Wellcome MS 213, Corlyon, p. 312.
15 Culpeper, *A Physical Directory*, p. 190.
16 The practice of smoking is described by Benjamin Woolley in *The Herbalist, Nicholas Culpeper and the fight for medical freedom*. London: HarperCollins, 2004, p. 22.
17 Wellcome MS 1071, Barrett, p. 112.
18 Wellcome MS 3107, Kidder, p. 268.
19 Thomas Dawson, *The Good Housewife's Jewel*. Lewes: Southover Press 1996 (From edition of 1596–7), p. 148.
20 Andrew Chevallier, *Encyclopaedia of Medicinal Plants*. London: Dorling Kindersley, 2001, p. 28.
21 Nicholas Culpeper, *Complete Herbal & English Physician* … J. Gleave & Son, 1826, p. 100.
22 Wellcome MS 213, Corlyon, p.158.
23 Pollington, *Leechcraft*, p. 393.
24 Tony Hunt, *Popular Medicine in Thirteenth Century England*. Cambridge: D.S. Brewer, 1990, p. 282. f. 40 r.
25 Wellcome MS 213, Corlyon, p. 159.
26 *ibid.*, p. 158.
27 *ibid.*, p. 280.
28 *ibid.*, p. 286.
29 *ibid.*, p. 288.
30 Grieve, *A Modern Herbal*, p. 422.
31 Wellcome MS 213, Corlyon, p. 286.
32 Hannah Woolley, *The Gentlewoman's Companion*. (Text of 1675.) Totnes: Prospect Books, 2001, p. 185.
33 W. M., *The Pearl of Practice*, p. 154.
34 Wellcome MS 213, Corlyon, pp. 188–9.
35 Stine, *Opening Closets*, p. 146.
36 Jacqueline Simpson & Steve Roud, *A Dictionary of English Folklore*. Oxford: Oxford U. P., 2000, p. 2. The example given is later, 1770, but the superstition may very well date back a long time.
37 W. M., *The Pearl of Practice*, p. 154.
38 Wellcome MS 3547, Miller, f. 74 r.
39 *ibid.*, f. 65 r.
40 Wellcome MS 213, Corlyon, p. 284.

CHAPTER 5: FEVERS AND FRETS

1   Porter, *The Greatest Benefit to Mankind*, p. 75.
2   Wellcome MS 213, Corlyon, p. 200.
3   *ibid.*, p. 189.
4   *ibid.*, p. 199.
5   Wellcome MS 774, Townsend, f. 15 r.
6   Markham, *The English Hous-wife*, 1615, p.5.
7   Markham, *The English Hous-wife*, 1631, p. 56.
8   Wellcome Ms 1071, Barrett, p. 11.
9   Wellcome MS 774, Townsend, f. 97 v. (Written in a large hand, suitable for an 'ancient body' to read.)
10   Wellcome MS 3547, Miller, f. 66 v.
11   Wellcome MS 213, Corlyon, pp 150–154.
12   *ibid.*, p. 249.
13   *ibid.*, p. 150.
14   Wellcome MS 1071, Barrett, p. 14.
15   Wellcome MS 1, Acton, f. 3.
16   Wellcome MS 213, Corlyon, p. 11.
17   Wellcome MS 3769, Parker, f. 67 r.
18   *Gerard's Herball*, ed. Woodward, p. 242.
19   *ibid.*, p. 201.
20   Wellcome MS 213, Corlyon, p. 10.
21   *ibid.*, p. 6.
22   W. M., *The Pearl of Practice*, p. 171.
23   *ibid.*, p. 171.
24   Wellcome MS 3769, Parker, f. 65 v.
25   Markham, *The English Hous-wife*, 1631, p. 21.
26   Wellcome MS 3547, Miller, f. 62 r.
27   Wellcome MS 213, Corlyon, p. 35.
28   *ibid.*, p. 33.
29   *Garard's Herball*, ed. Woodward, p. 201.
30   Wellcome MS 3769, Parker, f. 65 v.
31   W. M., *The Pearl of Practice*, p. 45.
32   Wellcome MS 213, Corlyon, p. 34.
33   Markham, *The English Hous-wife*, 1631, p. 19.
34   Wellcome MS 213, Corlyon, p. 51.
35   *ibid.*, p. 50.
36   Wellcome MS 1071, Barrett, p. 13.
37   Wellcome MS 3547, Miller, f. 69 r.
38   Markham, *The English Hous-wife*, 1631, p. 18.
39   *Gerard's Herball*, ed. Woodward, p. 120.
40   Wellcome MS 213, Corlyon, p. 199.
41   Markham, *The English Hous-wife*, 1615, p. 26.

42 *ibid.*, p. 25.
43 W.M., *The Pearl of Practice*, p. 77.
44 Culpeper, *A Physical Directory*, p. 178.
45 Wellcome MS 3769 Parker, f. 78 v.
46 Wellcome MS 213, Corlyon, p. 185.
47 Markham, *The English Hous-wife*, 1615, p. 34.
48 Woolley, *The Gentlewoman's Companion*, p. 184.
49 Grieve, *A Modern Herbal*, p. 179.
50 Drury, *Plant Lore in England*, p.166 onwards.
51 *Everybody's Pepys*, p. 40.
52 Wellcome MS 1071, Barrett, p. 26.
53 Wellcome MS 213, Corlyon, p. 59.
54 *ibid.*, p. 323.
55 Markham, *The English Hous-wife*, 1615, p.35.

CHAPTER 6: DESPERATE DISEASES: PLAGUE, POXES AND CONSUMPTION

1 Susan Scott and Christopher Duncan, *Return of the Black Death: The World's Greatest Serial Killer*. Chichester: John Wiley & Sons Ltd, 2004.
2 Simpson and Roud, *A Dictionary of English Folklore*, p. 295.
3 Stephen Porter, *The Great Plague*. Stroud: Sutton Publishing, 2003, p. 14.
4 Wellcome MS 213, Corlyon, pp. 166–172.
5 *ibid.*, p. 166.
6 *ibid.*, p. 169.
7 *ibid.*, p. 171.
8 *ibid.*, p. 168.
9 Markham, *The English Hous-wife*, 1615, p. 8.
10 *Everybody's Pepys*, p. 259.
11 Plat, *Delightes for Ladies*, p. 98.
12 Wellcome MS 3769, Parker, f. 68 v.
13 Gerarde, *The Herball*, p. 1075.
14 Wellcome MS 1071, Barrett, p. 18.
15 Cited in Bell, *The Great Plague in London*, p. 37.
16 *ibid.*, p. 158.
17 Peter Marshall, *The Philosopher's Stone*. London: Pan Books, 2001, p. 308.
18 Jacques Sadoul, *Alchemists and Gold*, trans. Olga Sieveking. London: Neville Spearman, 1972, p. 112.
19 Markham, *The English Hous-wife*, 1631, p. 10.
20 *The Closet of the Eminently Learned Sir Kenelme Digbie Kt. Opened* (1669), ed. Jane Stevenson and Peter Davidson. Totnes: Prospect Books, 1997, p. 122.
21 Markham, *The English Hous-wife*, 1615, p. 8.
22 Wellcome MS 3789, Parker, f. 69 r.
23 W. M., *The Pearl of Practice*, p. 31.
24 Wellcome MS 3769, Parker, f. 68 v.

25 Linda Pollock, *With Faith and Physic: The Life of a Tudor Gentlewoman, Lady Grace Mildmay 1552–1620*. London: Collins & Brown, 1993, p. 138.

26 Markham, *The English Hous-wife*, 1631, p. 50. He gives several other 'cures', another also containing mercury, and involving sweating.

27 *Selections from The History of the World Commonly Called The Natural History of C. Plinius Secundus*, translated by Philemon Holland, selected by Paul Turner. London: Centaur Press, 1962, [Book 28] p. 269.

28 Wellcome MS 213, Corlyon, p. 41.

29 Porter, *The Greatest Benefit to Mankind*, p. 452.

30 Culpeper, *A Physical Directory*, p. 17.

31 Woolley, *The Gentlewoman's Companion*, p. 184.

32 W. M., *The Pearl of Practice*, pp. 57–58.

33 Wellcome MS 213, Corlyon, pp. 77–78.

34 Cited in *The Occult in Early Modern Europe, A Documentary History*, edited and translated by P. G Maxwell-Stuart. Basingstoke and London: Macmillan Press, 1999, p. 125.

35 Culpeper, *A Physical Directory*, p. 50.

36 Wellcome MS 213, Corlyon, p. 90, which follows p. 79 in MS.

37 Wellcome MS 3547, Miller, f. 68 r.

38 Harvey, *The Family Physician*, p. 29.

Chapter 7: Diet, Digestion and Food as Medicine

1 Published about 1542.

2 *Andrew Boorde's Introduction and Dyetary … .* Woodbridge: Boydell & Brewer, 2000. Reprint of Early English Text Society ed. of 1870, p. 270.

3 *ibid.*, p. 271.

4 Translation published by Ente Provinciale Per il Turismo, Salerno, no date but twentieth century, pp. 22 and 66.

5 J.C. Cooper, *An Illustrated Encyclopaedia of Traditional Symbols*. London: Thames & Hudson, 1978, p. 66.

6 *Culpeper's Complete Herbal*, p. 356.

7 Markham, *The English Hous-wife*, 1631, p. 236.

8 *ibid.*, pp. 65–69.

9 Woolley, *The Gentlewoman's Companion*, pp. 169–170.

10 *ibid.*, p. 175.

11 Gerarde, *The Herball*, p. 325.

12 Wellcome MS 213, Corlyon, p. 316.

13 W. M., *The Pearl of Practice*, p. 149.

14 John Evelyn, *Acetaria, A Discourse of Sallets*. London: B. Tooke, 1699. Facsimile ed. London: Prospect Books, 1982, p. 89.

15 Wellcome MS 213, Corlyon, p. 115.

16 *ibid.*, p. 114.

17 W.M., *The Pearl of Practice*, p. 44.

18 Wellcome MS 213, Corlyon, p. 100.

19 Wellcome MS 3107, Kidder, p. 304.

20 Wellcome MS 213, Corlyon, p. 141.

21 *ibid.*, p. 144.

22 *ibid.*, p. 265.

23 *ibid.*, p. 146.

24 Wellcome MS 774, Townsend Family, f. 55 r.

25 Wellcome MS 213, Corlyon, p. 146.

26 Wellcome MS 3769, Parker, f. 76 r.

27 *Everybody's Pepys*, p. 70.

28 Culpeper, *A Physical Directory*, C 2.

29 Wellcome Ms 213, Corlyon, p. 138.

30 *ibid.*, p. 139

31 Woolley, *The Gentlewoman's Companion*, p. 185.

32 Gerarde, *The Herball*, p. 188.

33 *ibid.*, p. 398.

34 Woolley, *The Gentlewoman's Companion*, p. 197.

35 Wellcome MS 1071, Barrett, p. 38.

36 Culpeper, *A Physical Directory*, p. 50.

37 Wellcome MS 213, Corlyon, p. 122.

38 *ibid.*, p. 239.

39 Wellcome MS 3107 Kidder, p. 211.

40 Markham, *The English Hous-wife*, 1615, p. 34.

41 *Culpeper's Complete Herbal*, p. 71

42 Markham, *The English Hous-wife*, 1615, p. 31.

43 *Culpeper's Complete Herbal* p. 136.

44 Wellcome MS 213, Corlyon, p. 212.

45 Markham, *The English Hous-wife*, 1615, pp. 48–49.

46 Wellcome MS 213, Corlyon, p. 207.

47 *ibid.*, p. 209.

48 *ibid.*, p. 79.

49 *The Closet of ... Sir Kenelme Digbie*, p. 107.

50 *ibid.*, p. 109.

51 Dawson, *The Good Housewife's Jewel*, p. 135.

52 Markham, *The English Hous-wife*, 1615, p. 5.

53 Wellcome MS 213, Corlyon, p. 72.

54 Wellcome MS 3547, Miller, f. 33 v.

55 Wellcome MS 3107, Kidder, p. 77.

Chapter 8: Women and Children

1 Jane Sharp, *The Midwives' Book Or the whole Art of Midwifery Discovered*. New York & London, Garland Publishing, 1985. (Facsimile of edition of 1671), p. 129.

2   *ibid.*, pp. 250–251.

3   *ibid.*, p. 256.

4   Woolley, *The Gentlewoman's Companion*, p. 183.

5   Wear, *Knowledge & Practice in English Medicine*, p. 141.

6   Laurinda S. Dixon, *Perilous Chastity, Women and Illness in Pre-Enlightenment Art and Medicine*. New York: Cornell University Press, 1995, p. 241.

7   Wellcome MS 1071, Barrett, p. 135.

8   Gerarde, *The Herball*, p. 323.

9   Partridge, *The Treasvrie of Hidden Secrets*, chap. 74.

10   Warren R. Dawson, *A Leechbook or Collection of Medicinal Recipes of the Fifteenth Century*. (Text of MS 136, Medical Society of London.) London: Macmillan & Co. 1934, p. 124.

11   Markham, *The English Hous-wife*, 1631 p. 40.

12   Sharp, *The Midwives' Book*, p. 83.

13   *ibid.*, p. 76.

14   *Selections from Pliny*, p. 83.

15   Sharp, *The Midwives' Book*, p. 289.

16   *ibid.*, pp. 293–294.

17   Wellcome Ms 213, Corlyon, p. 197.

18   Sharp, *The Midwives' Book*, p. 242.

19   *ibid.*, pp. 239, 127.

20   Wellcome MS 1071, Barrett, p. 16.

21   *ibid.*, p. 82.

22   *ibid.*, p. 79.

23   John Graunt, *Natural and Political Observations &c.* in *A Collection of the Yearly Bills of Mortality From 1657 to 1758 inclusive*. London: A. Miller, 1759, p. 31.

24   Markham, *The English Hous-wife*, 1615, p. 32.

25   Partridge, *The Treasvrie of Hidden Secrets*, Chap. 90.

26   *ibid.*, Chap. 92.

27   Sharp, *The Midwives' Book*, pp. 164–165.

28   *ibid.*, p. 326.

29   Gerarde, *The Herball*, p. 389.

30   Deni Bown, *The Royal Horticultural Society's Encyclopaedia of Herbs & Their Uses*. London: Dorling Kindersley, 1995, p. 278.

31   Gerarde, *The Herball*, p. 1201.

32   Bown, *The RHS Encylopedia of Herbs*, p. 371.

33   Sharp, *The Midwives' Book*, p. 253.

34   Woolley, *The Gentlewoman's Companion*, p. 186.

35   Wellcome MS 1071, Barrett, p. 156.

36   W. M., *The Pearl of Practice*, p. 121.

37   Sharp, *The Midwives' Book*, pp. 253–254.

38   Graunt, *Observations etc.* p. 16.

39   Wellcome MS 1, Acton. f. 4.

40   Markham, *The English Hous-wife*, 1615, p. 32.

41 Sharp, *The Midwives' Book*, p. 208.

42 Gerarde, *The Herball*, p. 1072.

43 Markham, *The English Hous-wife*, 1631, p. 41.

44 Wellcome MS 1071, Barrett, p. 9.

45 Markham, *The English Hous-wife*, 1631, p. 39.

46 Woolley, *The Gentlewoman's Companion*, p. 179.

47 Wellcome MS 1071, Barrett, p. 5.

48 Wellcome MS 213, Corlyon, p. 65.

49 Sharp, *The Midwives' Book*, p. 213.

50 Wellcome MS 1071, Barrett, p. 62.

51 *ibid.*, p. 17.

52 *ibid.*, p. 62.

53 Sharp, *The Midwives' Book*, p. 408.

54 Grieve, *A Modern Herbal*, p. 816.

55 Wellcome MS 213, Corlyon, p. 54.

56 W. M., *The Pearl of Practice*, pp. 126–127.

57 Woolley, *The Gentlewoman's Companion*, p. 180.

58 W. M., *The Pearl of Practice*, p. 126.

CHAPTER 9: OLD AGE

1 Wellcome MS 213, Corlyon, p. 300.

2 *ibid.*, p. 311.

3 Wellcome MS 3107, Kidder, p. 263.

4 Wellcome MS 213, Corlyon, p. 194.

5 W. M., *The Pearl of Practice*, p. 108.

6 Gerarde, *The Herball*, p. 188.

7 Dawson, *The Good Housewife's Jewel*, p.146 and Wellcome MS 213, Corlyon, p. 302. It looks as if Mrs Corlyon had read Dawson, or perhaps they used a common source.

8 Dawson, *The Good Housewife's Jewel*, p. 147.

9 Gerarde, *The Herball*, p. 526.

10 Woolley, *The Gentlewoman's Companion*, p. 182.

11 Wellcome MS 213, Corlyon, p. 176.

12 Wellcome MS 3017, Kidder, p. 185.

13 Wellcome MS 213, Corlyon, p. 177.

14 *ibid.*, p. 309.

15 *Everybody's Pepys*, p. 225.

16 Wellcome MS 213, Corlyon, p. 266.

17 *ibid.*, p. 215.

18 *ibid.*, p. 129.

19 Wellcome MS 3769, Parker, f. 79 v.

20 Wellcome MS 1071, Barrett, p. 29.

21 Wellcome MS 3107 Kidder p. 229.

22 *ibid.*, p. 271.
23 Wear, *Knowledge & Practice in English Medicine*, p. 248.
24 Wellcome MS 213, Corlyon, p. 196.
25 *ibid.*, pp. 182 and 314.
26 Woolley, *The Gentlewoman's Companion*, p. 181.
27 Wellcome MS 3107, Kidder, p. 170.
28 Porter, *The Greatest Benefit to Mankind*, p. 270.
29 *Leaves from Gerard's Herball*, p. 109.
30 Wellcome MS 213, Corlyon, p. 246.
31 *ibid.*, p. 191.
32 Markham *The English Hous-wife*, 1615, p. 11.
33 W.M., *The Pearl of Practice*, p. 87.
34 Wellcome MS 3547, Miller, f. 54 v. - f. 55 v.
35 Harvey, *The Family Physician*, p. 131.
36 Wellcome MS 1071, Barrett, p. 128.
37 Wellcome MS 213, Corlyon, p. 51.
38 W.M., *The Pearl of Practice*, pp. 71–72.

CHAPTER 10: TROUBLED HEADS

1   Burton, *Anatomy of Melancholy*, vol. 1, p. 174.
2   See Carl Zimmer, *Soul Made Flesh: The Discovery of the Brain – and How It Changed the World*. London: Heinemann, 2004.
3   Wellcome MS 213, Corlyon , p. 303.
4   *Culpeper's Complete Herbal*, p. 210.
5   Wellcome MS 213, Corlyon, p. 19.
6   *ibid.*, pp. 22–23.
7   *ibid.*, p. 26.
8   *ibid.*, p. 23.
9   Markham, *The English Hous-wife*, 1631, p.11.
10 Wellcome MS 213, Corlyon, p. 21.
11 Markham, *The English Hous-wife*, 1631, p.17.
12 Sharp, *The Midwives' Book*, p. 330.
13 Wellcome MS 213, Corlyon, p. 17.
14 Burton, *Anatomy of Melancholy*, vol. 2, pp. 99–101.
15 Chevallier, *Encyclopaedia of Medicinal Plants*, p. 225.
16 Wellcome MS 213, Corlyon, p. 21.
17 *ibid.*, p. 22.
18 *Culpeper's Complete Herbal*, p. 281.
19 Harvey, *The Family Physician*, p. 133.
20 Markham, *The English Hous-wife*, 1615, pp. 34–35.
21 Gerarde, *The Herball*, p. 331.
22 *ibid.*, p. 1110
23 Burton, *Anatomy of Melancholy*, vol. 1, p. 175.

24   *ibid.*, p. 172.
25   Wellcome MS 1071, Barrett, p. 173.
26   *Leaves from Gerard's Herbal*, p. 166.
27   Gerarde, *The Herball*, p. 114.
28   Partridge, *The Treasvrie of Hidden Secrets*, chap. 122.
29   Gerarde, *The Herball*, p. 654.
30   Wellcome MS 213, Corlyon, p. 263.
31   *ibid.*, p. 152.
32   Wellcome MS 1071, Barrett, p. 225.
33   Ficino, *The Book of Life*, p. 20.
34   Burton, *Anatomy of Melancholy*, vol. 2, p. 120.
35   Markham, *The English Hous-wife*, 1615, p. 10.
36   Gerarde, *The Herball*, p. 190.
37   *ibid.*, p. 827.
38   *ibid.*, p. 357.
39   Markham, *The English Hous-wife*, 1615, p.10.

CHAPTER 11 : BEAUTY, COSMETICS, PERFUMES AND SOAP

1   John Evelyn, *Diary*, edited by Guy de la Bédoyère. Woodbridge: Boydell Press 1995, p. 87.
2   Pollock, *With Faith and Physic*, p. 125.
3   Wellcome MS 3769, Parker, f. 65 r.
4   Wellcome MS 3107, Kidder, p. 259.
5   *To make a very good Pomatum.* W. M., *A Queen's Delight*, p. 18.
6   *Everybody's Pepys*, 8 March 1664, p. 204. Pepys disapproved.
7   *ibid.*, p. 399.
8   W.M., *The Pearl of Practice*, p. 53.
9   Plat, *Delightes for Ladies*, p. 99.
10   Wellcome MS 3769, Parker, f. 66 r.
11   Partridge, *The Treasvrie of Hidden Secrets*, chap. 100.
12   *ibid.*, chap. 87.
13   *ibid.*, chap. 87.
14   Pollock, *With Faith and Physic*, p. 126.
15   Wellcome MS 3107, Kidder, p. 271.
16   W. M., *A Queen's Delight*, p. 105.
17   Partridge, *The Treasvrie of Hidden Secrets*, chap. 87.
18   Plat, *Delightes for Ladies*, p. 95.
19   Partridge, *The Treasvrie of Hidden Secrets*, chap. 106.
20   Markham, *The English Hous-wife*, 1615, p. 28.
21   Wellcome MS 3547, Miller, f. 23 r.
22   *Everybody's Pepys*, 27 March 1667, p. 382.
23   Culpeper, *A Physical Directory*, p. 231.
24   W. M., *A Queen's Delight*, p. 76.

25   W. M., *The Pearl of Practice*, p. 100.

26   William Turner, *Herbal*. Collen: Arnold Birckman, 1568 , Book I, f. 105 r.

27   Plat, *Delightes for Ladies*, p. 99.

28   W. M., *A Queen's Delight*, p. 77.

29   Partridge, *The Treasvrie of Hidden Secrets*, chap. 101.

30   Plat, *Delightes for Ladies*, p. 101.

31   Wellcome MS 1071, Barrett, p. 7.

32   Plat, *Delightes for Ladies*, p. 97

33   Dawson, *The Good Housewife's Jewel*, p. 151.

34   Partridge, *The Treasvrie of Hidden Secrets*, chap. 84.

35   Plat, *Delightes for Ladies*, pp. 91, 96.

36   *ibid.*, p. 63.

37   Wellcome MS 108, Baber, f. 2 r.

38   W. M., *A Queen's Delight*, p. 78.

Chapter 12: Magic, Superstition and Other Odd Ingredients

1   Monsieur Pomet and others, *A Compleat History of Druggs: Done into English from the Originals*. London: J & J. Bonwicke and others, 3rd edition, 1737, p. 257.

2   Pollington, *Leechcraft*, p. 239.

3   Hunt, *Popular Medicine in Thirteenth Century England*, p. 269 [f. 5 r.].

4   Wellcome MS 1073, Barrett, p. 28.

5   *ibid.*, p. 3

6   Wellcome MS 213, Corlyon, p. 249.

7   Dr Richard Mead, *Pharmacopoeia Pauperum*, 1718. Printed as a postcard by the Old Operating Theatre Museum and Herb Garret, St. Thomas's St., London SE1.

8   Wellcome MS 1073 Barrett, p. 44.

9   Harvey, *The Family Physician*, pp. 127 & 131. Incomes from Gregory King's Scheme, 1688, cited in Peter Laslett, *The World we have Lost*. London: Methuen, 1971, pp. 36–37.

10   Pomet, *A Compleat History of Druggs*, p. 234.

11   *ibid.*, p. 233.

12   Harvey, *The Family Physician*. There were alterations in price for bezoar stones in a list of errata. The final decision was a cost of 40s. the ounce for Oriental and 16s. the ounce for Occidental bezoar, p. 126 and errata page at back of book.

13   Wellcome MS 1073, Barrett, p. 233.

14   Markham, *The English Hous-wife*, 1615, p. 27.

15   Markham, *The English Hous-wife*, 1631, p. 14.

16   Wellcome MS 3107, Kidder, p. 273.

17   Culpeper, *A Physical Directory*, *Directions*, C verso.

18   Pomet, *A Compleat History of Druggs*, pp. 229–230.

19 Harvey, *The Family Physician*, p. 127.

20 Wellcome MS 213, Corlyon, p. 191.

21 Pollock, *With Faith and Physic*, p. 114.

22 Paracelsus, *The Archidoxes of Magic*, facsmile of English translation by R. Turner, London: Printed by J.C. for N. Brook and J. Harrison, 1656. London: Askin Publishers, & New York: Samuel Weiser, 1975, p. 117. Although attributed to Paracelsus this may be the work of the alchemist, Gerhard Dorn, originally written in 1570, or thereabouts.

23 Jane Stevenson & Peter Davidson, editors, *The Closet of the Eminently Learned Sir Kenelme Digbie*, Introduction, p. xxiii.

24 W. M., *The Pearl of Practice*, p. 181.

25 Burton, *Anatomy of Melancholy*, vol. 1, p. 255.

26 Sharp, *The Midwives' Book*, p. 106.

27 *ibid.*, p. 101.

28 *ibid.*, p. 208.

29 *ibid.*, pp. 354–355.

30 Porter, *The Greatest Benefit to Mankind*, p. 35.

31 *Selections from Pliny*, p. 275.

32 *The Greek Herbal of Dioscorides*, Englished by John Goodyer in 1655, but not printed until 1933. Oxford: Robert T. Gunther, 1934, p. 122.

33 Markham, *The English Hous-wife*, 1615, pp. 31–32.

34 Pollington, *Leechcraft*, p. 173.

35 *Selections from Pliny*, p. 276.

36 Wellcome MS 774, Townsend, f. 79 r.

37 Wellcome MS 1071, Barrett, p.116.

38 *ibid.*, p. 146.

39 W. M., *The Pearl of Practice*, 2nd ed., p. 192

40 Culpeper, *A Physical Directory*, p. 52.

41 *ibid.*, p. 54.

42 Wellcome MS 3107, Kidder, p. 192.

43 Paracelsus, *Archidoxes of Magic*, p. 93.

44 Wellcome MS 1073, Barrett, p. 156.

45 Culpeper, *A Physical Directory*, pp. 107–108.

46 *ibid.*, p. 239.

47 *ibid.*, p. 52.

48 *ibid.*, p. 120.

49 Pomet, *Compleat History of Druggs*, p. 400.

50 Culpeper, *A Physical Directory*, p. 53.

51 Pomet, *Compleat History of Druggs*, p. 402.

52 Cited in Joan Evans, *Magical Jewels of the Middle Ages and the Renaissance particularly in England*. New York: Dover Publications, 1976, p. 189.

53 Burton, *Anatomy of Melancholy*, vol. 1, p. 256.

Bibliography and Further Reading

Allen, David E. and Hatfield, Gabrielle, *Medicinal Plants in Folk Tradition: An Enthnobotany of Britain & Ireland*. Portland, Oregon and Cambridge: Timber Press, 2004.

Aubrey, John, *Brief Lives* ed. Richard Barber. London: The Folio Society, 1975.

Bell, Walter George, *The Great Plague in London*. ed. Belinda Hollyer. London: The Folio Society, 2001.

Bo[o]rde, Andrew, *The Fyrst Boke of the Introduction of Knowledge & A Compendyous Regyment of A Dyetary of Helth*. Early English Text Society, 1870. Woodbridge: Boydell & Brewer, reprinted 2000.

Bown, Deni, *The Royal Horticultural Society's Encyclopaedia of Herbs & Their Uses*. London: Dorling Kindersley, 1995.

Burton, Robert, *The Anatomy of Melancholy*. 3 vols. London: J. M. Dent, 1932. (First published 1621.)

Chevallier, Andrew, *Encyclopaedia of Medicinal Plants*. London: Dorling Kindersley, 2nd ed. 2001.

Cooper, J.C., *An Illustrated Encyclopaedia of Traditional Symbols*. London: Thames & Hudson, 1978.

Culpeper, Nicholas, *The English Physitian: Or An Astrologo-Physical Discourse of the Vulgar Herbs of the Nation*. London: Peter Cole, 1652.

——, *Culpeper's Complete Herbal*. London: Foulsham, no date.

——, *Culpeper's Complete Herbal, and English Physician* ... Barcelona: 1981. (Reproduced from an original edition published in 1826.)

——, *A Physical Directory Or a Translation of the Dispensatory Made by the Colledge of Physitians of London*. 2nd ed. London: Peter Cole, 1650.

Dawson, Thomas, *The Good Housewife's Jewel*. Lewes: Southover Press, 1996. (First published 1596–7.)

Dawson, Warren R. *A Leechbook or Collection of Medicinal Recipes of the Fifteenth Century*. (Text of MS 136, Medical Society of London.) London: Macmillan & Co., 1934.

Dioscorides, *The Greek Herbal of Dioscorides ... Englished by John Goodyer A.D. 1655*. Ed. and first printed 1933 by Robert T. Gunther. Oxford: University Press, 1934.

Dixon, Laurinda S., *Perilous Chastity, Women and Illness in Pre-Enlightenment Art and Medicine*. New York: Cornell University Press, 1995.

Drury, Susan Mary, *Plant Lore in England 1600–1800*. Unpublished M. Phil. Thesis, University of Leeds, 1984.

Evelyn, John, *Acetaria, A Discourse of Sallets*. London: Prospect Books, 1982. (Facsmile edition of 1699.)

——, *The Diary of John Evelyn*, ed. Guy de la Bédoyère, Woodbridge: The Boydell Press, 1995.

Evans, Joan, *Magical Jewels of the Middle Ages and the Renaissance, particularly in England*. New York: Dover Publications, 1976. (Reprint of Oxford: Clarendon Press edition, 1922.)

Ficino, Marsilio, *The Book of Life, A Translation by Charles Boer of Liber de Vita (or De Vita Triplici)*. Irving, Texas: Spring Publications, 1980.

Fraser, Antonia, *The Weaker Vessel: Woman's lot in seventeenth-century England*. London: Weidenfeld and Nicolson, 1984.

Gerarde, John, *The Herball or Generall Historie of Plantes*. London: John Norton, 1597. Amsterdam: Theatrum Orbis Terrarum, Facsimile 1974.

——, *Leaves from Gerard's Herball* ed. Marcus Woodward, London: Gerald Howe, 1931.

——, *Gerard's Herball: The Essence thereof distilled by Marcus Woodward*. London: Bracken Books, no date. (From the edition of Th. Johnson, 1636.)

Goodrick-Clarke, Nicholas, sel. & trans. *Paracelsus: Essential Readings*. Berkeley, California: North Atlantic Books, 1999.

Gregory, Andrew, *Harvey's Heart: The Discovery of Blood Circulation*. Cambridge: Icon Books, 2001.

Grant, Mark, *Galen on Food and Diet*. London: Routledge, 2000.

Graunt, John, *A Collection of the Yearly Bills of Mortality from 1657 to 1758 inclusive ... & Natural & Political Observations on the Bills of Mortality*. London: A Miller, 1759.

Grieve, Mrs M., *A Modern Herbal* ed. Mrs C.F. Leyel, Harmondsworth: Penguin Books, 1976.

Griggs, Barbara, *Green Pharmacy: A History of Herbal Medicine*. London: Norman & Hobhouse, 1981.

Harrington, Sir John, trans. *The School of Salernum: Regimen Sanitatis Salerni*. Salerno: Ente Provinciale Per Il Turismo, no date.

Hart-Davis, Adam, *What the Tudors & Stuarts Did For Us*. London: Boxtree, 2002.

Harvey, Gideon, *The Family Physician and the House Apothecary*. London: T.R., 1676.

Hatfield, Gabrielle, *Memory Widsom and Healing: The History of Domestic Plant Medicine*. Stroud: Sutton Publishing, 1999.

——, *Country Remedies: Traditional East Anglian Plant Remedies in the Twentieth Century*. Woodbridge: Boydell Press, 1994.

Henslow, G. *Medical Works of the Fourteenth Century together with a List of Plants recorded in Contemporary Writings* ... London: Chapman and Hall, 1899.

Hoffmann, David, *The New Holistic Herbal*. Shaftesbury: Element, 1986.

Hole, Christina, *The English Housewife in the Seventeenth Century*. London: Chatto & Windus, 1953.

Holmes, Frederick, *The Sickly Stuarts: The Medical Downfall of a Dynasty*. Stroud: Sutton Publishing, 2003.

Houdret, Jessica, *Pomanders, Posies and Pot-Pourri*. Princes Risborough: Shire, 1988.

Hunt, Tony, *Popular Medicine in Thirteenth-Century England: Introduction and Texts*. Cambridge: D.S. Brewer, 1990.

King, Helen, *Greek and Roman Medicine*. London: Bristol Classical Press, 2003.

Laslett, Peter, *The World we have lost*. London: Methuen & Co., 2nd ed. 1971.

Lee, Christopher, *1603: A Turning Point in British History*. London: Review, 2003.

Mann, John, *Murder Magic and Medicine*. Oxford: Oxford University Press, 1992

Markham, Gervase, *Countrey Contentments. The second Booke called the English Hous-wife* ... Amsterdam & New York: Da Capo Press, Theatrum Oribis Terrarum Ltd., 1973. (Facsimile of London editon of 1615)

——, *A Way to get Wealth* ... [Book 3] *The Office of the Housewife*. London: Nicholas Okes for John Harrison, 1631.

Marshall, Peter, *The Philosopher's Stone: A Quest for the Secrets of Alchemy*. London: Pan Books, 2002.

Maxwell-Stuart, P. G., Editor & translator, *The Occult in Early Modern Europe: Documentary History*, Basingstoke: Macmillan Press, 1999.

Moffat, Brian and others, *Sharp Practice 3, 4, 5, 6: Reports on Researches into the Medieval Hospital at Soutra, Scottish Borders* ... Edinburgh: Soutra Hospital; Archaeo-ethnopharmacological Research Project, 1989, 1992, 1995, 1998.

Pachter, Henry M., *Paracelsus: Magic into Science*. New York: Henry Schuman, 1951.

Paracelsus, *The Archidoxes of Magic: Of the Supreme Mysteries of Nature etc*. London & New York: Askin Publishers & Samuel Weiser, 1971 (First published in English in 1656.)

Partridge, John, *The Treasvrie of Hidden Secrets, Commonly called, The Good huswives Closet of provision, for the health of her Houshold*. London: Richard Oulton, 1637.

Pepys, Samuel, *Everybody's Pepys: The Diary of Samuel Pepys 1660–1669*, Abridged by O. F. Morshead. London: G. Bell and Sons, 1945.

Picard, Liza, *Elizabeth's London: Everyday Life in Elizabethan London*. London: Weidenfeld & Nicolson, 2003

——, *Restoration London*. London: Weidenfeld & Nicolson, 1997.

Plat, Sir Hugh, *Delightes for Ladies, To adorne their Persons, Tables, Closets and Distillatories* ... London: Crosby Lockwood, 1948. (From edition of 1609.)

Pollock, Linda, *With Faith and Physic: The Life of a Tudor Gentlewoman, Lady Grace Mildmay 1552–1620.* London: Collins & Brown, 1993.

Pollington, Stephen, *Leechcraft: Early English Charms, Plant Lore, and Healing.* Hockwold-cum-Wilton, Norfolk: Anglo-Saxon Books, 2000.

Pomet, Monsieur, and others. *A Compleat History of Druggs: Done into English from the Originals.* London: J. & J. Bonwicke and others, 3rd ed. 1737.

Porter, Roy, *The Greatest Benefit to Mankind: A Medical History of Humanity from Antiquity to the Present.* London: HarperCollins, 1997.

——, *Madness: A Brief History.* Oxford: Oxford University Press, 2002.

——, *Blood and Guts: A Short History of Medicine.* London: Allen Lane, 2002.

Porter, Stephen, *The Great Plague.* Stroud: Sutton Publishing, 2003.

Riddle, John M., *Dioscorides on Pharmacy and Medicine.* Austin: University of Texas Press, 1985.

Roud, Steve, *The Penguin Guide to the Superstitions of Britain and Ireland.* London: Penguin Books, 2003.

Sadoul, Jacques, *Alchemists and Gold.* Trans. Olga Sieveking. London: Neville Spearman, 1972.

Scott, Susan & Duncan, Christopher, *Return of the Black Death: The World's Greatest Serial Killer.* Chichester: John Wiley, 2004.

Sharp, Jane, *The Midwives' Book: Or the whole Art of Midwifery Discovered ...* New York and London: Garland Publishing, 1985. (Facsimile of edition of 1671)

Simpson, Jacqueline & Roud, Steve, *A Dictionary of English Folklore.* Oxford: Oxford University Press, 2000.

Sloan, A. W., *English Medicine in the Seventeenth Century.* Bishop Auckland: Durham Academic Press, 1996.

Stevenson, Jane & Davidson, Peter, eds., *The Closet of the Eminently Learned Sir Kenelme Digbie Kt. Opened (1669).* Totnes: Prospect Books, 1997.

Stine, Jennifer K., *Opening Closets: The Discovery of Household Medicine in Early Modern England.* Unpublished Ph. D. Dissertation, 1996. (Wellcome Library.)

Tobyn, Graeme, *Culpeper's Medicine: A Practice of Western Holistic Medicine.* Shaftesbury: Element, 1997.

Tomalin, Claire, *Samuel Pepys: The Unequalled Self.* London: Viking, 2002.

Turner, E. S., *Call the Doctor: a social history of medical men.* London: Michael Joseph, 1958.

Turner, Paul, sel. *Selections from The History of the World Commonly Called The Natural History of C. Plinius Secundus, translated into English by Philemon Holland.* London: Centaur Press, 1962. (Holland's translation originally published in 1601.)

Turner, William, *The first and second parts of the Herbal of William Turner.* Collen: Arnold Birckman, 1568.

Van de Weyer, Robert, sel. *Hippocrates: The Natural Regimen.* Berkhamsted: Arthur James, 1997.

W. M., *The Queen's Closet Opened: Incomparable Secrets in Physick, Chirurgery, Preserving Candying and Cookery; As they were presented to the Queen By the most Experienced Persons of the Times*. London: Nathaniel Brook, 1655,

——, *The Compleat Cook and A Queen's Delight* (Parts 2 & 3 of the whole work). London: Prospect Books, 1984. (Facsimile reprint of 1655.)

Wear, Andrew, *Knowledge and Practice in English Medicine, 1550–1680*. Cambridge: Cambridge University Press, 2000.

Wellcome MS 1. Acton, Grace. 1621.

Wellcome MS 108. Baber, Jane. *c.* 1625.

Wellcome MS 213. Mrs Corlyon. 1606.

Wellcome MS 774. Townsend Family. 1636–1647.

Wellcome MS 1071. Lady Barrett. *c.* 1700.

Wellcome MS 3107. Kidder, Edward & Katherine. 1699.

Wellcome MS 3547. Miller, Mrs Mary. 1660

Wellcome MS 3769. Parker, Jane. 1651.

White, Michael, *Isaac Newton: The Last Sorcerer*. London: Fourth Estate, 1997.

Woolley, Benjamin, *The Herbalist: Nicholas Culpeper and the fight for medical freedom*. London: HarperCollins, 2004.

Woolley, Hannah, *The Gentlewoman's Companion: or, A Guide to the Female Sex: The Complete Text of 1675*. Totnes: Prospect Books, 2001.

Zimmer, Carl, *Soul Made Flesh: The Discovery of the Brain – and How It Changed the World*. London: Heinemann, 2004.

Index

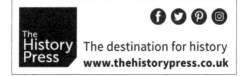